D0784451

'al

PATHS TO EMPOWERMENT

Edited by Marian Barnes and Lorna Warren

The POLICY
P~P
P R E S S

First published in Great Britain in 1999 by

The Policy Press
University of Bristol
34 Tyndall's Park Road
Bristol BS8 1PY
UK

Tel   +44 (0)117 973 8797
Fax   +44 (0)117 973 7308
E-mail tpp@bristol.ac.uk
http://www.bristol.ac.uk/Publications/TPP/

ISBN 1 86134 128 8

Marian Barnes is Director of Social Research in the Department of Social
Policy and Social Work at the University of Birmingham and **Lorna Warren**
is a Lecturer in Social Policy in the Department of Sociological Studies at the
University of Sheffield.

Cover design by Qube Design Associates, Bristol.
Printed in Great Britain by Hobbs the Printers Ltd, Southampton.

Contents

Notes on contributors

Marian Barnes is Director of Social Research in the Department of Social Policy and Social Work at the University of Birmingham. She has been engaged in research and development in the field of user involvement and user self-organisation for over 10 years. She acted as consultant to the Fife User Panels Project as well as coordinating the project evaluation. She has published widely in this area, including *Care, communities and citizens*, published by Longman in 1997.

Nina Biehal is a Senior Research Fellow in the Department of Social Policy and Social Work at the University of York. She has carried out research on young people leaving care and on user participation in social services and has also been involved in work on questions of welfare and citizenship for the Institute for Public Policy Research. She is currently involved in research on young people running away from substitute care.

Joyce Cormie has been a development officer with Age Concern Scotland for 10 years. In that time she has worked in a number of areas. Her first major piece of work, carried out at the behest of Fife Health Board and Fife Regional Council, was looking at aspects of day care within Fife. This led her to look into the needs of those suffering with dementia and their carers, and consequently she set up community dementia teams in three areas of Fife. Following on from this she implemented, with others, multi-agency training for those working in the field of dementia. She has been involved in the Fife User Panels Project from its inception in 1992 and continues to be actively engaged in this work, both within Fife and beyond.

Brian Davey trained as a development economist and has for many years been involved in the voluntary sector and community work in Nottingham. After several years of mental health problems, including many psychotic breakdowns, he became a development worker in the mental health field. From 1986 he played a role in the beginning of the user movement in Nottingham. He was otherwise initially chiefly concerned with different ways of understanding his own and other people's 'mental health' problems. Since 1990 he has been developing an environmental project to create new futures for users. He has also lived and worked in Germany at the Bauhaus Dessau Academy in 1996.

His book, *Strategy for outsiders*, will shortly be published in German translation by the Manz Schulbuchverlag Vienna. He has not had a psychiatric consultation since 1991.

Ken Davis is a disabled activist who became interested in disability issues a few years after an accident left him with a spinal injury while serving in the RAF in 1961. He is a founder member of a number of disability organisations including the Union of the Physically Impaired, DIAL UK, Derbyshire Coalition of Disabled People and the Derbyshire Centre for Integrated Living. A former miner and Labour councillor, he now lives in Clay Cross.

Alan France is a Research Fellow in the Department of Law at Sheffield University. His main interests are: the sociology of youth and childhood, citizenship and empowering methodologies. Over the previous three years he has written a number of articles that explore the meaning of citizenship for young people. He has also written about the role of development work and has co-authored articles that discuss the future of youth work in late modernity. His concerns in recent research have been with young people's beliefs about health, lifestyle and risk and he is presently writing about the relationship between health, citizenship and questions of masculinity and risk taking.

Lorna Warren is a lecturer in the Department of Sociological Studies at the University of Sheffield. She has been working on studies of community care since 1983. Her publications include *Changing services for older people* (1996), published by the Open University Press. She is currently working with older women in a research project which explores their health, image and lifestyles.

Adrienne Wright has been employed for over 20 years in the National Health Service, initially as a nurse, more recently as a manager. She has worked within various sectors including acute hospital services, acute community mental health services and services for older people. Having recently completed an MSc in Health Care Policy and Organisation at the University of Nottingham, she has taken up a full-time post as a manager within mental health services.

Introduction

Marian Barnes and Lorna Warren

Empowerment is one of the buzzwords of the 1990s. No respectable academic, policy or practitioner discourse is complete without its nod in the direction of the empowered consumer, the empowered citizen, or even the empowered worker. It is easy to become cynical when repetition of the language of empowerment seems to substitute for substantial change in practice. But the very frequency with which the term appears within such discourses should tell us something. If it is not always a reality in practice, it may be a real aspiration for many of those committed to a renewal of the relationship between public services and their users. We are sufficiently optimistic to suggest that real shifts in understanding are taking place and that new voices are being heard in contexts from which they have formerly been excluded. In policy and practice areas as diverse as social security provision (Swift et al, 1994), health service purchasing (Smithies, 1996) and individual mental health needs assessments (Bristol Social Services/South West MIND, nd) and many more, it is possible to identify practical examples of the way in which participative approaches to decision making are becoming familiar, if not normal, practice. The contributors to this collection all have their reservations about the extent to which that represents a real shift in the balance of power. They would also question whether the crafting of more empowered 'customers' really addresses the most important issues in the lives of those who have often been defined by their relationship with welfare services. But all recognise that there are opportunities to be taken in an environment in which the rhetoric of empowerment has reached places in which it was not previously heard. While they are realistic about what can be achieved working within systems and structures which have not been designed with empowerment as an objective, nevertheless they recognise, as Brian Davey writes, that "if we start small enough we can get started".

Our practice as researchers and teachers *is* being influenced by those new voices, even if we sometimes struggle to learn new ways of working and new ways of relating to those with whom we work in these capacities. We invite service users to contribute to teaching on social work or social policy courses, but do we invite them to contribute to determining the curriculum for these courses? And if we try to do so, how can we accommodate this along with all those other bodies we have to satisfy regarding content and standards? As researchers, we welcome people stepping out of the respondent role to take their place in determining research questions to be explored. But when it comes to crafting the articles through which we hope to disseminate research findings how many of us are still working alongside those we have been researching? And when we are dependent on winning grants from funders requiring detailed research proposals which set out methods, criteria and timetables in advance, how can we convince them to take what appears to be the more risky option of developing participatory approaches which require agreement to be reached at all stages about how to proceed?

Perhaps more fundamentally, how successful have we been in developing research strategies which are based in disabled people's experiences of social exclusion, in young people's experience of alienation from the world of work, in older people's sense of being regarded as a non-productive burden on those in work, or in the stigma which comes with the label of mental illness? While it is no longer difficult to get research funding to explore the views of young people about strategies intended to divert them from crime, or the views of older people about health services (see France and Cormie in this collection), the agenda is still being dominated by the concerns of service commissioners or providers. User groups themselves are increasingly carrying out research into users' views of services (see, for example, Beeforth et al, 1994), but few are in a position to carry out or commission research which addresses the type of issues identified by Brian Davey or Ken Davis in their papers in this collection.

The seminar series from which these papers are drawn, and which was entitled 'Alliances and Partnerships in Empowerment', was intended to address some of the issues and dilemmas faced when those who might formerly have occupied different places within service and knowledge systems seek to establish new types of relationship with each other. As workers within a university department committed to research which can have an impact in the world of policy and practice, we sought to bring together those active in empowerment projects, and those who study such projects, to discuss and debate what we have all learnt from those experiences. We aimed to provide a forum in which people could openly debate ideas and experiences in a way which might reflect the participative process necessary to the achievement of individual and collective empowerment, as well as contribute to the development of new understanding and knowledge.

The experience of these seminars demonstrates some of the issues to be faced in seeking to develop new relationships of this type. Administratively and financially it was easiest for us to invite people into the university, rather than to organise seminars in community locations with which participants might be more familiar. Taking our cue from the way in which the Greater London Council under Ken Livingstone opened up the doors of County Hall to the Londoners who were governed from within it, we also wanted to open up the university to people who might have regarded this as an environment from which they were excluded. But did that inhibit people from attending? There was only one occasion on which 'users' outnumbered 'academics' and on that occasion transport had been arranged to bring groups of disabled people together.

And what about the format of the seminars? We aimed to ensure there was plenty of opportunity for discussion, in small groups as well as when people were all together, but is the idea of asking one person to 'give a paper' that is then discussed something that we assume is a useful approach because that's what we are familiar with? Would we have done better in terms of sharing experiences and seeking to develop shared understandings if we had invited a number of people to come and tell their stories, rather than putting one person in the limelight?

With these questions in mind, we followed up the seminar series with an event which was intended to build on the initial links which had been made. The occasion was a workshop which was called 'Working in Partnership' (Warren, 1997) and had five key aims:

- to identify barriers to effective working between service users; carers; service purchasers and providers; and academics;
- to explore how those barriers might be overcome;
- to identify practical examples of projects on which groups might work together;
- to identify who should be involved in such projects;
- to consider how to take these ideas further.

Future goals which we had in mind included carrying out research together, and involving users and carers in teaching and training, as well as in service planning and development.

The workshop was a day-long event, held in a day centre that was chosen because it was reasonably close to Sheffield city centre and more likely to be territory familiar to users and carers. The numbers of participants were limited for practical and strategic reasons. Unfortunately, by this stage the resources earmarked for the development of 'Alliances and Partnerships in Empowerment' activities were running low. At the same time, however, we were recognising that for some individuals, who were not used to discussing their experiences or airing their views publicly, speaking in front of a large number of people might act as a deterrent to their (full) participation. Invitations were therefore issued to attenders of previous seminars, though special efforts were put into encouraging participants from a range of users and carers, including those from minority ethnic groups who had been notably absent from the seminar series[1], and, likewise, from people working in a range of positions within health and social services, as well as the voluntary sector. It is interesting to note that users and carers collectively outnumbered the latter, though there was a relatively good turn out by academics/ researchers.

The event was led by an independent facilitator, Jonathan Swift, who had experience of being an informal carer as well as having worked as a professional in both health and social care services (as a nurse and a social worker), and of working in a university department. Jonathan steered participants through the muddy waters of health and social care policy, highlighting recent changes which have been of most salience to the notion of user and carer empowerment. However, it was through his establishment of a series of small-group discussions on 'barriers' and 'assistances' (sic) to user and carer involvement in services that he achieved a much more free-flowing debate than had been previously generated within the seminar series. Tape recordings of randomly chosen groups revealed a process of 'story-telling' (Bertaux, 1981; Cotterill, 1992) taking place on the part of all respective participants (see Warren's paper in this collection for further discussion of some of the issues raised). The closing debate on ways forward for partnerships suggested that the desire, certainly on the part of users and carers, was not necessarily directly to attack professional roles per se but rather to demystify them. The challenge for professional organisations (especially the health services) was to make clearer the various different bodies involved in decisions affecting users' and carers' lives. Above all, different organisations needed to be brought together more effectively, on the one hand to open up channels of communication and avoid inflexible assessments of need and provision of services and their wasteful duplication and, on the other, to prevent 'buck-passing' and Eurocentric, service-led responses to need which led to people 'falling through the net'. The call was not for users and carers to take over professionals' roles (including researching needs), but rather to ensure that their activities were directed by user and carer interests and value-bases.

Our aim in this series of seminars and workshops was to discover ways in which researchers and teachers, people who use services, and people who provide services could develop better understanding of each other's interests, concerns and skills and more effectively work together in partnership. The objectives of such partnerships were perceived as contributing to the empowerment of young people, older people, disabled people and others who have been cast as 'clients' of welfare services. We were not entirely successful in building bridges between the different worlds of those in 'academia', those who purchase and provide services, and those who use services. But even in distinguishing between those three groups we were aware that such categorisations are not always real: we are all potential users of services, even when we are also service providers or university workers, and self-interest alone might be considered sufficient reason to develop alliances. This is most clearly the case in relation to health services where everyone is likely to come into contact with services at some stage in their lives. Nevertheless, it is also important to understand the real power differences that exist between those who occupy positions within organisations controlling the resources through which welfare is delivered, and those who seek access to those resources. The urgency of health and social care needs can generate a frustration with those who seek long-term changes through incorporating the lessons from research in service planning and training of future health and social care workers. We are continuing to explore ways in which we might better understand what can be the benefits of working in partnership.

In planning the seminar series and inviting people to contribute to it we did not start from any one theory or model of empowerment. For all the groups represented here, the issue of empowerment in relation to health and social care services is only one aspect of their experience of disempowerment and exclusion. This comes over clearly in the papers by Brian Davey and Ken Davis. The paper by Ken Davis has been updated to include reflection on more recent policy debates which are causing considerable concern among disabled people. Campaigns among disabled people for anti-discrimination legislation are part of a broader campaign for equal citizenship which are still far from being realised. But even if we consider empowerment in relation to services, the way in which people *use* services varies considerably and models or routes to empowerment are correspondingly varied (Barnes and Prior, 1995). For example, empowering people to become more active participants in decision making in relation to whether or not to have an operation (Meredith, 1993) is likely to be rather different from that involved in engaging young people in the process of investigation of suspected child abuse (Roberts and Taylor, 1993). Thus how people define and understand the process of empowerment is likely to be affected by their experiences of themselves in relation to society as a whole, as well as by the circumstances and conditions in which they make use of services.

It became evident from the papers presented here, and from the discussions they generated, that one major dilemma is the very different meanings associated with the term 'empowerment'. Our starting point was a deliberately broad notion of empowerment as embracing the opportunities for people to become more influential both in determining the nature of the services they receive, and in exercising control over their lives as a whole (Barnes and Walker, 1996). In the context of altering the balance of power between providers and users of services, we sought to recognise the need for change in openings for users to develop skills necessary to participation, as well as in the practice of workers. While much of the discussion of the latter is based on the experiences of research workers, the tensions and potentialities involved in developing new approaches to the practice of research have a resonance for workers in other contexts seeking to develop partnership practice. Adrienne Wright's paper describes the experience of someone appointed to a mental health trust to develop 'user involvement'. She soon realised that it was necessary to undertake development work with staff as well as with users if real change in the way in which services were to be provided was to be achieved. In the concluding paper in this collection Lorna Warren addresses some of the different ways in which empowerment has been understood, and how empowerment (or the lack of it) may be understood by the different groups participating in the seminar series.

In preparing the papers for publication they have not been edited to make them conform to one view of empowerment, nor to one type of language in which aspirations towards empowerment may be expressed. Nor have we asked people to conform to the conventions of academic writing which typically draws on other literature to support arguments (as in this introduction!). Ideas and analyses which come from reflections on lived experiences are central to the development of new knowledge and understanding about empowerment. New voices may be uncomfortable to hear: both because of what they have to say and the way in which this is expressed (Barnes and Wistow, 1994). As Joyce Cormie makes clear, the development of listening skills is central to the success of any project which seeks to include those rarely heard when important decisions about services are being made. And as Brian Davey demonstrates, those whose horizons are constrained by the organisational context in which they work may be made uncomfortable by the ideas of 'losers' who have no investment in existing structures. Ken Davis reflects on the way in which discomforting ideas which challenge existing power structures may be resisted through being transformed into something else: civil rights and citizenship become a need for 'care'. Thus we have not attempted to edit papers in a way that is intended to make them conform to a particular notion of an appropriate discourse within which such ideas should be expressed. Marian Barnes herself appreciated the significance of this when one of her papers was 'copy-edited' in preparation for publication in another collection. The paper concerned Marian's relationship with a group of carers with whom she was working on a research project. It explored the nature of the relationship that developed and how this shaped the research process and made possible insights which would not have been obtained from a research relationship in which the researcher is required to maintain distance from her 'subjects'. The copy-editor transformed a piece written in the first person to the third person and effectively undermined the whole purpose of the paper until s/he was asked to undo the editing.

The practice of research has itself been subject to scrutiny for its potential to empower or disempower (eg, Beresford, 1992; Barnes, 1993; Reason, 1994; Fetterman et al, 1996). Users of welfare services have themselves pursued research as one strategy to achieve their aims and have challenged professional control over research in the same way that they have challenged professional control over services (eg, Oliver, 1987; Davis, 1992; Beeforth et al, 1994). One particularly disempowering aspect of traditional research practice has been the typically exclusive focus of researchers on the technical aspects of the process and a failure to consider its 'social' aspects. Related to this has been a fear of admitting in print that things did not quite work out as planned. The credibility of research has been assumed to depend on the researcher being completely in control of the process, an assumption which has contributed to its elite status and which bears very little relation to the often messy reality of research in practice.

More reflective approaches to research are being encouraged, not least as a result of the contribution of feminist researchers (eg, Roberts, 1981; Stanley and Wise, 1983; Warren, 1990), and the potential for research to contribute to the empowerment of excluded groups has been recognised in new approaches to the conduct of research (eg, Shakespeare et al, 1993; Reason, 1994; Fetterman et al, 1996). Nevertheless, other influences, such as the domination of scientific models of research within key funding agencies and the pressure to produce 'academic' articles to support promotion prospects, act to limit the capacity of those employed in professional capacities as researchers to implement methods more capable of empowering those involved in the research. Lorna Warren develops some of the reasons for this in her paper. User groups, community groups and others not recognised as 'researchers' often find it difficult to obtain funding to undertake their own projects, although, as Viv Lindow demonstrated in a later paper in this seminar series, the Joseph Rowntree Foundation has sought to shift the balance somewhat by funding research in which users are active participants (Lindow and Morris, 1995).

In this collection three researchers, Marian Barnes, Nina Biehal and Alan France, reflect on ways in which they have attempted, not always successfully, to do research *with* rather than *on* people. None would claim that the approaches they adopted are representative of 'empowerment research', but they do demonstrate ways in which researchers can start to make a difference and they demonstrate a preparedness on the part of researchers to admit to their difficulties in developing more participatory ways of conducting research. The contributors to this collection continue to seek to find paths to empowerment based on inclusive methods of working. We hope this collection will encourage others to do the same.

Note

[1] We would like to thank Nell Farrell for the part she played in ensuring that positive efforts were made to recruit participants from minority ethnic groups and to acknowledge that the audience was, nevertheless, still composed predominantly of white participants.

References

Barnes, M. (1993) 'Introducing new stakeholders: user and researcher interests in evaluative research. A discussion of methods used to evaluate the Birmingham Community Care Special Action Project', *Policy & Politics*, vol 21, no 1, pp 47-58.

Barnes, M. and Prior, D. (1995) 'Spoilt for choice? How consumerism can disempower public service users', *Public Money and Management*, vol 15, no 3, pp 53-8.

Barnes, M. and Walker, A. (1996) 'Consumerism versus empowerment: a principled approach to the involvement of older service users', *Policy & Politics*, vol 24, no 4, pp 375-93.

Barnes, M. and Wistow, G. (1994) 'Learning to hear voices: listening to users of mental health services', *Journal of Mental Health*, vol 3, pp 525-40.

Beeforth, M., Conlan, E. and Graley, R. (1994) *Have we got views for you. User evaluation of case management*, London: Sainsbury Centre for Mental Health.

Beresford, P. (1992) 'Researching citizen involvement: a collaborative or colonising exercise?', in M. Barnes and G. Wistow (eds) *Researching user involvement*, Leeds: Nuffield Institute for Health, University of Leeds.

Bertaux, D. (ed) (1981) *Biography and society: The life history approach in the social sciences*, London: Sage.

Bristol Social Services/South West MIND (nd) *The Avon Mental Health Measure. A user-centred approach to assessing need*, Bristol: South West MIND.

Cotterill, P. (1992) 'Interviewing women: issues of friendship, vulnerability and power', *Women Studies International Forum*, vol 15, no 5/6, pp 593-606.

Davis, A. (1992) 'Who needs user research? Service users as research subjects or participants: implications for user involvement in service contracting', in M. Barnes and G. Wistow (eds) *Researching user involvement*, Leeds: Nuffield Institute for Health, University of Leeds.

Fetterman, D.M, Kaftarian, S.J. and Wandersman, A. (eds) (1996) *Empowerment evaluation. Knowledge and tools for self-assessment and accountability*, Thousand Oaks: Sage.

Lindow, V. and Morris, J. (1995) *Service user involvement: Synthesis of findings and experience in the field of community care*, York: Joseph Rowntree Foundation.

Meredith, P. (1993) 'Patient participation in decision-making and consent to treatment: the case of general surgery', *Sociology of Health and Illness*, vol 15, no 3, pp 315-36.

Oliver, M. (1987) 'Re-defining disability: some implications for research', *Research, Policy and Planning*, vol 5, no 1, pp 9-13.

Reason, P. (ed) (1994) *Participation in human enquiry*, London: Sage.

Roberts, H. (ed) (1981) *Doing feminist research*, London: Routledge and Kegan Paul.

Roberts, J. and Taylor, C. (1993) 'Sexually abused children and young people speak out', in L. Waterhouse (ed) *Child abuse and child abusers*, London: Jessica Kingsley.

Shakespeare, P., Atkinson, D. and French, S. (eds) (1993) *Reflecting on research practice: Issues in health and social welfare*, Buckingham: Open University Press.

Smithies, J. (1996) *Community participation in health purchasing: A review of examples of interesting practice*, Haworth: Labyrinth Training and Consultancy.

Stanley, L. and Wise, S. (1983) *Breaking out: Feminist consciousness and feminist research*, London: Routledge and Kegan Paul.

Swift, P., Grant, G. and McGrath, M. (1994) *Participation in the social security system*, Aldershot: Avebury.

Warren, L. (1990) *Doing, being, writing: Research on home care for older people*, Feminist Praxis, monograph number 31.

Warren, L. (1997) *Alliances and partnerships in empowerment: The 'Working in Partnership' Workshop*, Unpublished report, Sheffield: Department of Sociological Studies, University of Sheffield.

Part One

Definitions, models and practice

Introduction to Part One

While the 1980s and 1990s saw the development of top-down initiatives to promote user involvement and consumer empowerment, this period also saw a substantial increase in the self-organisation of people who had previously been constructed as clients of welfare services. These new 'user groups' are different from many traditional voluntary organisations operating within the welfare sphere and, indeed, some have their origins in opposition to voluntary organisations claiming to act 'for' disabled people and others, without being directly controlled by the people they claimed to represent. Groups have formed around identities such as the shared experience of being in local authority care: the National Association of Young People in Care (NAYPIC); of experiencing mental health problems: Survivors Speak Out, MINDLINK and the UK Advocacy Network (UKAN); of having a learning difficulty: People First; of being disabled: the British Council of Disabled People; of being older and in receipt of state pensions: the National Pensioners' Federation; and of looking after a friend or relative: the Carers' National Association.

Organisationally such groups are highly diverse. Many groups are solely locally based and exist primarily to provide support and information to members at a local level. They are often dependent on the enthusiasm of particular individuals and are highly vulnerable to any change in circumstances. Others have secured funding and have been able to employ a few staff, at least on short-term contracts. But they, too, are vulnerable to changes in policy among funders and may find their activities constrained by the nature of the funding available. They may find themselves torn between wanting to influence 'from the inside' – through direct involvement in planning or contracting, for example – and adopting an independent position as both collective and individual advocates. Some groups are affiliated to national umbrella organisations and aim to influence national policy and the education and training of welfare professionals. Together they constitute a social movement with a significance extending beyond the immediate impact of changes to be achieved in particular local services. Both activists and analysts have compared this 'user movement' with other action for social change pursued within women's movements, among black people and among gay and lesbian people.

The importance of distinguishing the objectives of autonomous user groups from those of officials seeking to recruit users to action controlled from within agencies has also been emphasised. While the development of a consumerist ideology within public services provided a legitimation for user influence, both the forms and objectives of such influence are contested. In particular, the way in which knowledge is constructed and contributes to the power of welfare professionals over those who use services has been the subject of contestation between user groups and researchers, as well as between such groups and service providers. Increasing control over knowledge production is seen as a key part of the strategy of many groups actively engaged within the movement.

The contributions to this part of the collection provide examples of different ways of thinking about the world which have developed within parts of the user movement and which challenge many professional assumptions. Ken Davis, from within the disabled people's movement, and Brian Davey, starting from the experience of having been diagnosed with a mental illness, provide perspectives on the meaning of 'empowerment' which are at odds with the way the term is used within many professional discourses. Joyce Cormie worked as a development worker with Age Concern Scotland when she was involved in establishing the Fife User Panels Project. Her contribution provides an example of a voluntary organisation *for* older people seeking to ensure the voices being heard are those *of* older people. Her chapter also discusses the discomfort of some professionals when faced directly with older people in the role of 'questioners' rather than as passive recipients of expert knowledge. Adrienne Wright's contribution considers some of the dilemmas faced when those within health and social care agencies acknowledge the differences of perspectives and priorities among users, but have to operate within 'the system' to achieve a change in the practice of health workers.

These contributions can only provide illustrations of the different, and sometimes conflicting, voices to emerge from within the user movement and from among voluntary and statutory sector allies. Below, we list other texts which discuss similar issues and which interested readers may wish to follow up.

the building of the welfare state, Hunt (1992) notes that the development of disability as an administrative category under the Poor Law is seen by Stone not only in terms of controlling eligibility for the provision of welfare, but also exemption from certain obligations of citizenship:

> **In the regulations of Poor Law administration and thus in the eyes of Poor Law administrators, five categories were important in defining the internal universe of paupers: children, the sick, the insane, 'defectives' and the 'aged and infirm'. Of these, all but the first are part of today's concept of 'disability'. Everyone else was defined able-bodied by default. (Stone, 1984, p 40)**

Indeed, after the Poor Law was amended in 1834, the majority of workhouse inmates were in fact "... physically and mentally disabled, the aged, the orphan and a wide variety of sick" (Wood, 1991, pp 98-9). As a result, disabled people were socially stigmatised by a system that was designed first and foremost as a deterrence to the able-bodied.

The Poor Law officials were the forerunners of today's social services professionals, and it was in their interest of course to perpetuate their own administrative role. The extent of their success can be judged by the fact that, with amendments, the system endured for three and a half centuries until it evolved into the welfare state, just after the Second World War. The passage of the welfare state's safety net, the 1948 National Assistance Act, moved Aneurin Bevin to declare that the Poor Law was at last buried, showing how wide the gap between rhetoric and reality can often be. Certainly, Parliament had repealed the Poor Law on paper but it retained in practice some of its most time-hallowed elements, not least among which in Part III was its predilection for incarcerating disabled people in institutions and then obliging them and their families to pay towards the cost of being segregated from the community. And of course, it was also careful to retain the administrative approach to disability for the new post-war generation of welfare officials.

Within this administrative tradition, the departmental officials who dreamed up 'community care' policy in the 1960s would have done so as naturally as their 17th-century predecessors did when they coined the phrase 'outdoor relief' to describe their policy of providing Poor Law help outside the workhouse. No account was taken of the discontent with the lack of community-based alternatives to institutional provision which was growing among disabled people at that time. The struggles of disabled people to escape from, or reform the running of, segregated residential institutions during the 1960s, using first-hand knowledge of the shortcomings of the system, were not significant in the official mind. Given their Poor Law legacy, their views and aspirations were seen as of no consequence.

Turning the controlling tide

Against this background, there was little choice for disabled people other than to try and bring change in a more determined and organised way. The main medium through which this struggle for social change has found expression has been organisations set up and run by disabled people, initially as a reaction against the conditions of life that have been thrust upon them and then proactively, redefining disability as a socially constructed phenomenon, analysing and identifying the social barriers that prevented participation in the mainstream and taking action on solutions. Finally, their organisations have taken to the streets in pursuit of civil rights and other, related, legislation that would do something to gain a measure of control over their lives.

The reactive process of challenging those who were controlling disabled people's lives started towards the end of the last century with organisations like the British Deaf Association (BDA) and the National League of the Blind (NLB). In the same way that trade unions were forming to improve and protect the economic and social position of working people, so were these organisations concerned to improve the lot of people who were deaf and blind. The NLB registered as a trade union in 1899, no doubt informed and inspired by the workers' movement in much the same way that civil rights struggles elsewhere fuelled the later stages of disabled people's self-organisation here in Britain.

These early organisations run by disabled people tended to seek improvements very much in the prevailing welfarist mode. The new deterrent Poor Law system had begun to crack under the strain of the economic, social and medical needs thrown up by industrialisation, and a number of self-help and charitable organisations had emerged in response. Some ran workshops, paying only a pittance to disabled workers, and the NLB was set up by blind workers in such places. Given the various welfare enactments which came at the end of the 19th century in the areas of education, pensions and national insurance, it would have seemed natural to the newly emerging disabled people's organisations to pursue improvements in that mould.

Indeed, bringing pressure for more or better welfare characterised disabled people's organisations until the situation changed with the formation in the early 1970s of the Union of the Physically Impaired against Segregation. This group paved the way for a civil rights struggle when it redefined disability as

> **... the disadvantage or restriction of ability caused by a contemporary social organisation which takes little or no account of people who have physical impairments and thus excludes them from participation in the mainstream of social activities. (UPIAS, 1976, p 14)**

By this 'social model' approach, UPIAS pointed the way out of the cul-de-sac in which disabled people's bodies were blamed as being the source of their problems. For the first time, socially created disability was charged with being a particular form of social oppression which could be overcome only by disabled people themselves taking the lead in a struggle for social change. It was a stage in development that grew rapidly from the early 1980s, with the emergence of many new organisations controlled by disabled people. Notable among these was the Disabled People's International (DPI) which was formed by disabled people, as Driedger (1989) describes, in response to the rejection by the disability professionals who ran Rehabilitation International (RI) of a motion which called for them to share power in RI equally with its disabled members.

In 1981, the British Council of Disabled People (BCODP) was formed and became Britain's representative body on DPI through its regional framework, and this in turn gave rise to a flood of member organisations controlled by disabled people around the country. This whole worldwide network is underpinned by the social model of disability, united in Britain around the need for anti-discrimination legislation in the form of a comprehensive and enforceable Civil Rights Bill, and its member organisations work in a variety of ways to remove the social barriers which prevent the full participation of its members as equal citizens in mainstream social life.

The clash of opposing ideas

Shakespeare sees this growth of activity among disabled people in the broader context of late 20th-century 'new social movements' engaged in the struggle for genuine participatory democracy, social equality and justice, which have arisen out of the crisis in industrial culture

(Shakespeare, 1993). Armed with its social model of disability and demand for equal citizenship, this movement was on course for a confrontation with the established controllers of disability policy from the very beginning.

During the 1980s, while the previous Conservative government was grappling along with many industrial societies, with the problem of restructuring state welfare, the disabled people's movement was painstakingly building up through its democratic organisations a very different campaign for civil rights. Predictably enough, this quickly ran into opposition, given the clash of opposing ideas. An early taste of the blunt use of power came when the government rejected the recommendation of the Committee on Restrictions against Disabled People (CORAD) that "there should be legislation to make discrimination on the grounds of disability illegal" (Large, 1982, p 53). Some 14 further rejections followed until an attempt to kill a Labour member's Civil Rights Bill in 1994 went so badly wrong that the Tories were embarrassed into bringing in the 1995 Disability Discrimination Act (DDA). Their hostility to the idea that disabled people should enjoy the same rights and share the same opportunities equally with everyone else is reflected in the Act's medical definitions, limited scope, allowances for 'justified discrimination', and poor provisions for implementation and enforcement. Accordingly, it encountered wholesale rejection by the disabled people's movement and its supporters.

On community care, it was not until it encountered a critical Audit Commission (1986) report that the Tory government got down to thinking about legislation. The latter was followed by the Griffiths Report (DHSS, 1988) and, in due course, by a White Paper, *Caring for people* (DHSS, 1989). During this process there was some consultation with the newly emerging disabled people's organisations. The Audit Commission (1986) report drew a critical response from BCODP (1987) and Sir Roy Griffiths met some disabled people's organisations as he prepared his report. By comparison with the influence wielded by vested interests outside the disabled people's movement, however, these consultations made very little impression on the essential features of the legislation when it eventually followed in the shape of the 1990 NHS and Community Care Act.

In the administration of the new Act, the Tories had been persuaded that local authorities should continue as successors to the power first given to them over four hundred years before in 14 Eliz 1572, an Act "for the punishment of vagabonds and the relief of the poor and impotent" (Fisher and Jurica, 1977, pp 590-8). It was interesting to see this Elizabethan conjunction of punishment and care reflected in Tory measures designed to punish so-called welfare fraudsters and layabouts within their own overall plans for the restructuring of state welfare. However, in Tudor England, times were different inasmuch as they waited until you were a pauper before the authorities intervened – today social services departments have the power to intervene, then turn disabled people into paupers through assessments, means tests and charges for residential or community care.

Thus the controlling ethos of social services remained intact, as did their medical model basis of community care. To be sure, community care may deploy some of the rhetoric of the disabled people's movement: independence, choice and control together with buzzwords like user empowerment are common enough in Guidance and other documents. And indeed, a nod toward the existence of the movement can be discerned in the requirement on local authorities to involve 'users' in planning. But the practice is still dominated by administrative concerns, and the overall effect has led Finkelstein (1997) to consider that the version of community care currently on offer is

> **.. a pernicious influence in maintaining the boundary between disability and normality, just at a time when disabled people are challenging the artificiality of this and other boundaries that constrain our, and non-disabled people's, lifestyles. (Finkelstein, 1997, p 13)**

Throughout the years of disabled people's self-organisation and collective struggle, what has been most fundamentally amiss boils down to two main issues. First, a limpet-like attachment by the disability establishment to a 'medical model' view of disability; second, the disproportionate distribution of power and influence between those who control disability policy and disabled people themselves. The weight of policy and practice still largely rests on the backward but convenient tradition of assuming that disabled people are different, with special needs and that their dependence requires the intervention of properly trained people who care and provide for them. This contrasts with the weight of policy and pressure in the disabled people's movement which is based on the conviction that all people are vulnerable and interdependent, and that we all have needs which are best catered for in a society which celebrates difference, which guarantees everyone's rights and freedoms, and which supports and provides equal opportunities for everyone to participate in everyday human affairs.

Resolving tensions

The desire of the Conservative government to impose 'care' was much stronger than any wish to confer on disabled people the kind of ordinary civil and social rights which, were they denied to the non-disabled population, would give rise to widespread social unrest. In 1997, new Labour came to power at the May elections and with the change came an unfamiliar wave of hope and optimism for the future. However, it soon seemed as though Labour's support for civil rights in opposition had weakened now they were in power. There was no trace of it in the Queen's Speech, nor even a mention of Britain's six million or so disabled people, many of whom had voted Labour into office. Labour's new Ministerial team contained no one with Cabinet status having sole responsibility for disability affairs. Instead, it was tagged on to a Junior Minister's employment brief, apparently as a bit of an afterthought.

This brought back and heightened the distrust stemming from seemingly endless years of Tory hostility towards civil rights, and it was not until the close of 1997 that some confidence, albeit cautious, began to be restored. Labour's Minister for Employment and Disability Rights, Andrew Smith MP, then started to act on promises made in his Conference speech earlier in the year of a Task Force to consider how best to secure comprehensive, enforceable civil rights for disabled people within the context of wider society, and to make recommendations on the role and functions of a Disability Rights Commission. However, the extent to which legislation might occur within the lifetime of the present Parliament may well depend on the movement's capacity to build support and maintain pressure on the government. Much less doubtful is that the DDA, warts and all, is here to stay for some time, perhaps until Labour has worked out its wider rights programme which includes the incorporation of the European Convention on Human Rights into UK law.

At the start of 1998, new tensions arose not just because of the slow progress on comprehensive civil rights legislation, but also over the intentions of new Labour on welfare reform. The focus in the opening weeks of the new year was on Labour's review of disability benefits, an element of state welfare which, in disabled people's experience, is clearly in need of reform. Under Labour, the hope was that this task would be undertaken positively but the opening gambits suggested that a crude cost-cutting exercise was afoot and that, in order to fulfil its election pledges, the government was simply seeking to find money where it felt it was likely to meet the least resistance. On community care, one of the last gasps of the outgoing Tory government, under pressure from the disabled people's movement, was to introduce legislation allowing local authorities to make direct payments which would enable disabled people to pay for and control their own personal assistance needs. Such direct payments are discretionary, the eligibility criteria are tight and social services departments still assess, decide how much and control the conditions under which the cash is doled out. There is thus much room for improvement since the disabled people's movement regards the right to independence and the resources needed to enable them to live full and productive lives as a fundamental human rights issue. However, at the time of writing, the detail of Labour's overall policy on disability benefits and community care in relation to its Welfare to Work proposals and within its wider rights agenda was unclear.

The need to resolve the tensions arising from such uncertainties has become as important to government popularity as it is for disabled people. The social model of disability demands an holistic approach to disability policy and a social welfare system which is geared to support it. Finkelstein and Stuart have speculated about the kind of services that might emerge if social model principles informed the facilities needed by disabled people. In their view, such a future system would need to ditch the medical model 'cure or care' approach in favour of provisions which recognise disabled people's rights, and empower and enable them to control their own lives. Such a system would

> **... be conceived in terms of 'support' and would acquire an enabling role in the same way that public utilities (eg postal services, railways, water and electricity supplies, etc) are created by able-bodied people for able-bodied people to enable more satisfying lifestyles. As such, they (would) form part of the necessary public support network which enabled both full participation in society and citizenship rights. (Finkelstein and Stuart, 1996, p 171)**

Where the new Labour government stands on such matters remains to be seen and, at this stage, disabled people are not anticipating very many radical changes in basic assumptions about the nature of the problems they face. They are aware that the disability industry has gathered a lot of power in the four centuries or so of its development since the Old Poor Laws. They are aware that powerful vested interests, both political and professional, calculate that they have more to gain from keeping disabled people dependent than from liberating and supporting their independence. The political climate may be changing, but the battle for disabled people's citizenship rights remains to be won.

References

Audit Commission (1986) *Making a reality of community care*, London: HMSO.

BCODP (British Council of Organisations of Disabled People) (1987) *Comment on the Audit Commission's Report 'Making a reality of community care'*, Summary on the Report of the Audit Commission, London: BCODP.

DHSS (1988) *Community care: An agenda for action. A report to the Secretary of State for Social Services* (Griffiths Report), London: HMSO.

DHSS (1989) *Caring for people: Community care in the next decade and beyond*, London: HMSO.

Driedger, D. (1989) *The last civil rights movement: Disabled Peoples International*, London: Hurst & Co.

Finkelstein, V. (1993) 'Disability: a social challenge or an administrative responsibility?', in J. Swain, V. Finkelstein, S. French and M. Oliver (eds) *Disabling barriers – Enabling environments*, London: Sage Publications, in association with the Open University.

Finkelstein, V. (1997) 'From enabling to disabling, an open university?', Valedictory Lecture, The Open University, Milton Keynes.

Finkelstein, V. and Stuart, O. (1996) 'Developing new services', in G. Hales (ed) *Beyond disability: Towards an enabling society*, London: Sage Publications.

Fisher, H.E.S. and Jurica, A.R.J. (eds) (1977) '14 Elizabeth, c. 5, Statutes of the Realm, IV, Part I', in *Documents in English economic history, England from 1000 to 1760*, London: G. Bell & Sons Ltd.

Hunt, J. (1992) 'The disabled people's movement between 1960-1986 and its effect upon the development of community support services', Unpublished MA dissertation, Leeds: University of Leeds.

Large, P. (1982) *Report by the Committee on Restrictions against Disabled People*, London: HMSO.

Shakespeare, T. (1993) 'Disabled people's self-organisation: a new social movement?', *Disability, Handicap and Society*, vol 8, no 3, pp 249-64.

Stone, D. (1984) *The disabled state*, London: Macmillan.

UPIAS (Union of the Physically Impaired against Segregation) (1976) *Fundamental principles of disability*, London: UPIAS.

Wood, P. (1991) *Poverty and the workhouse in Victorian Britain*, Stroud: Alan Sutton Publishing Ltd.

The Fife User Panels Project: empowering older people

Joyce Cormie

Introduction

Age Concern Scotland (ACS) is a voluntary organisation which seeks to represent the interests of older people to policy makers. As an organisation it has recognised the importance of ensuring that the views it represents are genuinely those of older people, rather than what staff think those views might be (Age Concern, 1993). The project described in this chapter was designed to enable older people themselves to have their say about community care. It focuses on older people who make considerable use of community care services and who thus are unlikely to be active members of Pensioners' Forums or other organisations which have developed to represent older people's views directly.

The Fife User Panels Project was developed because it became evident to us in ACS that the 1990 NHS and Community Care Act requirement on social services departments to listen to the voice of users of services in planning and providing community care services was not happening as far as very frail older people were concerned. This gap was particularly significant since elderly people are probably the greatest users of services. Equally we recognised that reaching out to this population of frail, mostly housebound, people could prove extremely difficult. Averil Osborn, then Assistant Director of Age Concern Scotland, and I began to examine ways of engaging older people in discussions about the future direction services should be taking.

One principle we felt must be key to our work in developing this project was the central place of older people themselves (Age Concern Scotland, 1992). We set up an Advisory Group involving three older women as well as ACS project workers. Subsequently, after funding was received, we added representatives from local health and social work agencies. This group made a most significant contribution while we were setting up the project. They were involved in finalising the proposals which were submitted to Charity Projects, who funded the initiative, and in the selection of the resource worker. They have continued to play a valuable role as the Project has progressed but sadly one member died during the course of the project.

The Fife User Panels Project was initially funded for three years. The work commenced in October 1992 with the first panel being set up in March 1993 (Age Concern Scotland, 1992). Seven panels were established throughout the region during the three-year period (Age Concern Scotland, 1992) and have continued to meet beyond this initial project period. After Charity Projects funding ran out, local health and social work agencies agreed to provide continuing support for this work.

Figure 1 is a copy of a leaflet which outlines the purpose and nature of the project. This was given to home carers, district nurses, social workers and others who might be able to suggest members for the panels, and to older people who expressed interest in joining.

Figure 1: The Fife User Panels Project

WHAT is the project?
Panels set up to give older people an opportunity to express their views, needs and experiences and develop ways in which they can influence community care services.

WHY are we doing this?
* As a response to the changes happening in the way care services are provided by social work, health board and others.
* To discuss with older people how they see their needs and how they would like these to be met.
* To feed older people's views into the planning process to ensure that they are being considered.

HOW will this be done?
* Groups of six to eight people will be invited to meet locally for an hour or two for discussion with the two project workers.
* Transport will be arranged to and from the meeting place.
* The panels will meet in the afternoons, approximately every six weeks.
* The meetings will be in an easily accessible, comfortable room where tea, coffee etc. will be provided.

WHO will be asked to participate?
A cross-section of older people. However, we particularly want to include housebound older people who are not part of clubs or other networks and who are seldom asked their views. All those attending can be assured of the confidentiality of what they say.
* * * * * * * * * * * * * * * * *
We realise we are asking a lot of people but we hope these meetings will be a pleasant afternoon for all who attend.

USER PANELS PROJECT

	Joyce Cormie	Fife Development Officer
AGE	Maureen Crichton	Resource Worker
CONCERN	Jessie Watt	Secretary
SCOTLAND	152 High Street, Kirkcaldy,	
	Fife KY1 1NQ	
	Telephone: 01592 204273	

The overall purpose of the panels may be familiar to those with an interest in user involvement in community care. In this paper I want to concentrate on how we have sought to achieve this.

Groups of six to eight older people are invited to attend local meetings to have discussions with my colleague and me. We have to find a really comfortable setting for them. The vast majority of the panel members cannot get out of their own homes without special transport so that has to be arranged. This includes minibuses with hydraulic tail lifts, taxis, and my colleague and me collecting people in our cars. Meetings last for two hours with a break halfway through for tea/coffee. It is important to make it an enjoyable afternoon for the panel members, without too long a journey. We aim for no one having to travel for longer than 20 minutes. Of course the venues for the meetings have to be accessible – we have to make sure that there are no stairs and that there is access for wheelchairs as well as toilets accessible to disabled people. The original idea was that meetings would take place every six weeks. The members of the original Advisory Group felt it would suit older people better to have these meetings occurring at more regular times and so on their advice we increased the frequency of meetings to monthly.

Keeping the numbers at six to eight has required recruiting additional members from time to time. This has been because some members were no longer physically able to come because of illness or admission to residential care and because, sadly, some died during the course of the project. A good core of original members remained throughout the three-year project period, but recruiting new members has been a continual process and has taken more time than we had originally anticipated.

Who are the panel members?

The aim has been to involve people who are over 75 years of age, who are living alone, who are unable to get out without some form of support and who are in regular receipt of services. In most cases our members are quite heavy users of services and the vast majority live alone. We have members in their 90s but the majority of those coming are in their mid to late 80s. We feel in terms of involving older people we are meeting our target (Barnes et al, 1994).

People are nominated to join the panels in a variety of ways. Most nominations come about as a result of meetings with groups of practitioners in health and social services and with key people in the voluntary sector. We tell them about the purpose of the project and explain to them the criteria for panel membership. We were struck that from time to time remarks were made by professionals to the effect that:

"You'll never get these old folk to talk, they don't know what they need."

"You don't need to ask them, that is what we are trained to do, we know what all their needs are."

"They won't be capable of discussing things with you."

I must say we were pretty appalled at these attitudes!

Ways of working

Panel meetings initially involve just sitting and chatting, at least that is what it sounds like – just chatting. But we are talking with the panel members about where they come from, what sort of circumstances they are living in, what life is like for them at the moment, exploring what they did in the past, finding out what they enjoyed doing that they can no longer do and gently, gently considering their background and their life now. The panel members set the agenda and topics raised early in the discussions included such things as transport and safety in the home. Soon conversations begin to get into issues more specifically related to health and social care services.

Not surprisingly, changes in the home care service have prompted extended discussions in all the panels. For the recipients of these services there have been quite dramatic changes in our area (and probably throughout the UK) and our members have observed a move away from a home help service to that of personal care. As one empowered panel member said two years down the line to a senior social worker "You never discussed it with us when you decided to change the policy!"

The home help topic provides a useful illustration of the way we work with the panel members. Once the importance of the home help services had emerged from conversations if we had asked the panel members what they thought about their home help you can imagine that 99% of them would say, "She's wonderful", "great", "just like a daughter" etc. Instead we started from a different point. We asked the older people to examine the needs within their home – what tasks they couldn't do themselves and would require to be done by someone else, how often they required these tasks to be done, and the priority with which they required the tasks to be done. We listed these in that manner on flip chart paper. We then looked at what the current home help service could and could not provide by examining with panel members the social work department's *Home carers handbook*. From that, we began to get a picture that the things that are done by home helps were often the things that many older people could do themselves and the things that are not being done are the very things the panel members said had highest priority: washing windows, changing curtains, putting in replacement light bulbs, for example.

There are a variety of ways in which we proceed once we have collected this type of information. Sometimes we will collate all the material collected from the different panels and send it to the person responsible in the region or one of the assistants in an area (we are working in three distinct social work areas). The older people will invite the appropriate person to a panel meeting to explore a bit more how some of their needs could actually be taken on board. This is what happened in relation to the home help issue.

One issue which emerged from discussions about home help services was the question of service charges. At the time, Fife prided itself, quite rightly, on its policy of giving free home help services. There are many other services provided free of charge in Fife such as Crossroads and the Alzheimer Sitter Service. Interestingly, when we started exploring with the panel members how some of their needs could be met they actually introduced the idea that they could perhaps pay for specific tasks. They have come up with various other solutions to some of the problems, including establishing a voluntary sector-run service to undertake tasks which could not be done by council-employed home helps. We are trying to promote such ideas at a regional level – we are getting there but it takes time to see significant changes.

Sometimes the discussions will result in the panel members asking for more information, more explanations, or offering their views in resolving some of the problems they have discussed. From time to time they will invite the relevant person from the social work department, the health board or other public agency to come and discuss matters further with them. This did not happen right away; it was about a year before the first panel to be established felt comfortable with the idea of someone coming to the group. It has been interesting for us to observe those invited from the social and health agencies to attend the meetings. The first thing that strikes my colleague and me is how nervous they often are. You can see that these professionals are not all at ease sitting down and meeting six or seven frail older people. It is a very unfamiliar setting for them to be in (which probably says a lot about the previous planning process), and many of the professionals do appear to feel extremely uncomfortable to begin with.

One of the ways they try to overcome this feeling is to arrive armed with their own agenda. For example, when the home help service manager came to meet with the panel on the first occasion we had sent one side of A4 paper highlighting some of the issues which had been discussed. We do this with all the people who are invited to give them a feel about the topics likely to be raised. This home help manager sat down and said to me, "Right Joyce, where do you want me to start?" I had to say that he hadn't quite got the point of the meeting. It appeared that he viewed the notes as a checklist and that he intended to go through this to tell the panel members why they couldn't get the services they wanted. For him and for others it has been quite a challenge for them to realise that this is not what the meetings are about and that they have to start listening and become involved in a dialogue with the panel members. Subsequently this manager attended panel meetings on three occasions and he began to relax and to value what the older people have to say.

As the panels have developed, the statutory agencies are beginning to have more and more knowledge of them and actively to seek out panel members' views. We will not take such requests to the panel meetings unless it is appropriate – in other words it has some definite linkage with what members have previously raised themselves. One request to the panels came from Fife Healthcare Trust asking for responses to the design of a questionnaire exploring their understanding of how older people's health needs are met within the community. The older people analysed everything – the cover, the colour, the illustrations, the type of print, the actual questions, the content of the questions, the appropriateness of the questions, and queried things which they did not understand. For example, in the questionnaire there was a margin with little squares with no explanation of what these were for. There had already been instructions about ticking one set of boxes, so what where these other little boxes all about? There was no indication that these were for the purpose of analysis and should be ignored by those completing the questionnaire. There were questions panel members felt were very intrusive, so they wanted to know who exactly got this information and what they would do with it. The result of that whole piece of work was that Fife Healthcare went back to the drawing board and rewrote the questionnaire. They then sent it out in the form that was acceptable to the panel members. It went to a thousand homes in

Fife of people over 75 years of age, and they received a 70% return, which in any research terms is pretty good. When things like that happen people begin to see the value of actually engaging older people in the process.

Another example of statutory agencies seeking input from the panels was when Fife Health Board were anxious to know what information was coming out from the panels about GPs, experiences in hospital and similar topics. Again we explained that the agenda was determined by members and that we would not ask the older people directly about this. As information in these areas came up we would start collating it. Over a period of 18 months we were able to collate from the different panel meetings observations made on a whole range of health issues such as experiences of GPs, hospital discharge, access to physiotherapists, occupational therapists, the ambulance service and so on. We then wrote a paper and circulated it to Fife Health Board, Fife Healthcare Trust (responsible for priority and community care in Fife) and the social work department.

One aspect of that paper involved a very specific look at hospital discharge based on some pretty awful personal experiences of the panel members. They shared these experiences with each other and started identifying things that shouldn't have happened, but which appeared to be fairly common. Since our aim is to use panel members' experiences to seek improvement in services we always try to get the panel members to turn their negative experiences into something positive. In the case of hospital discharge when they were telling about some bad experiences they themselves would say what should have happened or others would say what they would have expected from a good quality service. From this the panels, jointly, came up with a 14-point good hospital discharge checklist. An article on panel members' views about hospital discharge was published in the *Health Service Journal* (Barnes and Cormie, 1995). The older people were pointing out very basic requirements which would ease the experience of discharge, such as the house being warm, the need for services to be in place on the day of discharge, one hot meal being ready. They ended up regretting the passing of the almoner in hospitals whom they saw as a wonderful person (usually a woman) who made sure that everything was going to be all right when they got home. Of course that has the implication that there should be a key worker responsible for coordinating arrangements.

Interestingly, that whole batch of health-related papers has sparked off a tremendous amount of interest, again raising the profile of the panels, making people realise that there is virtue in talking to the members of the panels in looking at where things should be going in the future. The hospital discharge checklist has provided the focus for a multi-agency working group established to review existing procedures with a view to improvement.

A learning process

We are all learning together through this project but there is still a lack of understanding about the nature of the panels. It is hard for service providers to understand that the starting point for panel discussions is the experiences of older people themselves, rather than the concerns of those responsible for services. The purpose of the panels is to enable older people to be proactive rather than reactive. For example, we were asked if the panel members would respond to a leaflet which was to be given to older people who had to go into day hospital. What we got was the leaflet in draft form, which we felt immediately restricted the discussion to what was actually written down. We would have expected them to have come to the older people and said, "We are going to do a leaflet and want to know all the things that you would want to know before you go into hospital". In other words, giving them a blank sheet. Of course they might miss things out, but the starting point should be what older people themselves say they need to know, rather than what those who are providing the day hospital care feel they need to know.

As the panels have progressed it has become easier to engage in early consultation between the panel members and those responsible for services. For example, the regional manager for older people in the social work department regularly attends various panel meetings as well as meeting the project workers on a regular basis in order to find out what is coming out of the panels. As a result she can continuously feed information into community care planning rather than once a year as occurred previously.

These developments are very encouraging but there are still problems about the way the older people are addressed and considered by the service planners and providers. Some of the latter appear a bit scared but others are somewhat condescending and a bit patronising. One of our panel members was feeling a bit despairing about such attitudes and said, "Do they think we have just arrived from Mars?" On another occasion I was rather short with a visitor from the Health Board who had not done his homework and did not seem to know what the panels were all about. I was a little taken aback when one panel member said, after he had gone, "You were a bit hard on him, Joyce." However, another panel member said, "No, I think you were quite right. I think he thought he was coming just to patronise a group of old ladies".

Similarly, after the panel members had commented on the social work complaints procedure leaflet, a member of the Client Relations Office came to a panel meeting to discuss this further. Rather than discussing panel members' comments about the leaflet she proceeded to tell panel members how they could go about making a complaint. They were not at all pleased with her. They were terribly polite at the time of her visit but afterwards they were really annoyed, "We weren't asking her how to use the complaints procedure, we were complaining about the complaints procedure!"

These experiences demonstrate how unfamiliar it is for many professionals working in health and social care services to engage in direct dialogue with older people who use their services. Everyone is in a learning mode, but it is probably the professional people who come into the meetings, rather than the older people who are panel members, who have to make the biggest adjustments. Professionals have to look afresh at their working practices.

Two years into the project we held a conference where we brought together panel members, planners, service providers and researchers. We are always determined that the panel members will be on equal terms with whoever is visiting and so it was with this conference. It was an excellent day of exchanging ideas, listening to each other, having misconceptions challenged, all on the most egalitarian terms. We had workshops involving similar numbers of panel members and statutory personnel. Where possible we also tried to keep members of the same panels together. On the whole they were with the people they knew and they were radiating confidence.

One example illustrates the value of the direct contact enabled by such events. In the group I was facilitating there were representatives from the Health Board, the Healthcare Trust and the social work department, along with six panel members. At one point the Health Board person gave information about a service and said, "Of course you will all know about it". She was referring to a telephone 'Healthline' which is a way of trying to reach out to people who are not aware of, or happy with, elements of the health service in Fife. But the panel members all sat there and said, "No, we haven't heard of it". This was responded to with, "You must know about it. It is in our Newsletter which goes to every house in Fife". It was interesting to see people from statutory agencies realising that the information from their agencies was not reaching out in the way they assumed. Information is an issue which comes up frequently at panel meetings: the lack of information; poorly expressed information; wrongly targeted information; information coming at the wrong time. There seemed to be an assumption by service providers that because they had gone through their bit of the process, somehow at the other end people are absorbing this information and are ready to use it when required. They needed to hear directly from panel members that the information they were disseminating was not reaching its intended target.

There is an increasing willingness among professional staff to work with the panel members in determining service quality and standards. Nevertheless, some still find it difficult to accept that people they often regard as inarticulate and dependent are able to assert their needs and experiences so clearly. While the conference was highly valued by all who attended, one or two service providers suggested that the older people who attended were not "the same as the people that we deal with!". However, many said at the end of the conference that it had been the most wonderful day they had had at work for years. They were very excited and felt it was something that should be kept as a regular event.

User panels – a route to empowerment?

By the end of the three-year project period the value of the panels had become widely recognised and the User Panels Project was written into the strategy plans of Fife Health Board, Fife Healthcare NHS Trust and Fife social work department. As the evaluation of the project has shown (Barnes and Bennet-Emslie, 1997; Barnes and Bennett, 1998), panel members have valued the experience of being involved and in some areas it is possible to point to issues on which they have made an impact in terms of services. Does this mean that the panels have enabled the older people to become empowered? Have we been doing something that allows them to act differently? My first thought would be that these people are not actually any different when they are attending the panel meetings than they would be if they were meeting over a cup of coffee anywhere else – so I have to think again about 'empowerment'. I try to analyse what we are doing and I think one of the main things is that we are listening. Sometimes, when people are coming in to talk with the panel members you can see that they are not always listening, but waiting to get in with their bit and hence not hearing what people are actually saying and picking up cues.

We also aim to ensure the panel members can learn from those who come to meet the panels. We sometimes have to ask people invited to panel meetings to speak more accessibly. When they are using unfamiliar words or initials we will say, "Do you mean ..." and they realise what they are doing and stop using jargon. Both listening and speaking clearly are essential to effective dialogue.

Another characteristic of the panels which can be considered to contribute to a process of empowerment is that we follow the older people's agenda. It is true that now they are responding to work put to them but that is because they want to do it and it is always on issues or topics they have already explored. Even when we are looking at specific pieces of written work coming from service agencies the panel members determine how they are going to approach this. For instance, when we were talking about the content of the information for day hospitals leaflet the first thing it said was, "You will be picked up by ambulance at 8.30 am and you will arrive at the day hospital at 9.30 am". Now that was a statement of fact but the panel members discussed this at some length, pointing out that 8.30 am was far too early for most of them to be ready and that this early collection time could be a 'turn off' for potential attenders. That was relayed to those who had asked for comments. So we are following the older people's agenda – we are taking everything they say seriously.

We acknowledge the value of anecdotal material and I think that is very, very important. Anecdotes are ways of expressing personal experiences and of opening up the possibility of sharing those experiences with others. They provide a way into identifying both similar and different experiences and of reflecting on ways of making sense and responding to them. There is much to be learnt from the way in which people recount what has happened to them and it would be wrong to dismiss such accounts as 'mere anecdotes'.

Finally, working with older people in a way which might be considered to be 'empowering' cannot be achieved if those involved hold ageist attitudes. When we go in to panel meetings, we are sitting with friends – it is very enjoyable and it is a lot of fun. It is a process which we think has generated considerable value both for ourselves as project workers and for the older people who have been and continue to be involved.

References

Age Concern (1993) *Recognising our voices*, London: Age Concern England.

Age Concern Scotland (1992) *Fife User Panels Project: Seminar report*, Kirkcaldy: Age Concern Scotland.

Age Concern Scotland (1994) *New ways of working: First report to charity projects, October 1992-September 1993*, Edinburgh: Age Concern Scotland.

Age Concern Scotland (1995) *Forging new links: Report of Fife User Panels Conference*, Edinburgh: Age Concern Scotland.

Barnes, M. and Bennet-Emslie, G. (1997) '*If they would listen...*', An evaluation of the Fife User Panels, Edinburgh: Age Concern Scotland.

Barnes, M. and Bennet, G. (1998) 'Frail bodies, courageous voices. Older people influencing community care,' *Health and Social Care in the Community*, vol 6, no 2, pp 102-1.

Barnes, M., Cormie, J. and Crichton, M. (1994) *Seeking representative views from frail older people*, Edinburgh: Age Concern Scotland.

Barnes, M. and Cormie, J. (1995) 'On the panel', *Health Service Journal*, 2 March, pp 30-1.

Solving economic, social and environmental problems together: an empowerment strategy for losers[1]

Brian Davey

This paper is about 'a strategy for losers'. What I mean by this is an empowerment strategy for groups who come last in society. It is a strategy for putting the last first. I am referring here to two types of 'last' social groups. First, groups concentrated in particular localities and neighbourhoods because poverty and social disadvantage tend to be highly concentrated in geographical areas. Second, groups defined by one of a variety of social disadvantages that tend to limit and exclude equal consideration and equal resource availability in society: for example, racism, disability, a mental health diagnostic label and so on.

Conventional economic policies are based on the idea that we should all strive in competition either as individuals to get a job or to attract the favour of powerful economic interests. The aim of local economic policy is to attract inward investment from big employers into areas of poverty in competition with other areas. But it is in the very nature of competition that there are losers and when there are an increasing number of areas and people in the world who are losers this attempt to join the mainstream ceases to be credible. This is why I devised this title, 'a strategy for losers'. It is an attempt to find a different way forward.

People who are seriously disadvantaged in society rarely have single problems – they have multiple interlocking problems. They do not compete on a level playing field. They suffer a 'cycle of deprivation'. Empowerment must address all their problems together if it is to be meaningful. Poverty, poor housing and the nature of the social security system put a strain on relationships and lead to widespread demoralisation. Depending on the circumstances of individuals they can lead to physical and mental ill health, criminality, addiction and the persecution of individual or collective scapegoats: racism, sexism, picking on individuals who are 'different'. Disadvantaged people usually can only afford to live in areas where there is poor air quality, low car ownership but heavy traffic and other inferior environmental conditions – particularly those which pose a danger to children and thereby add to the stress of their parents.

Powerlessness has economic, environmental, social, interpersonal, health, emotional and cognitive dimensions. Powerless people live in limiting physical surroundings; they are spatially and socially separated from the people and places who decide about their destiny; they are not 'well connected'; they have lower purchasing power as consumers, no purchasing power for entrepreneurial and investment roles and they are often emotionally and cognitively crippled by powerlessness – either not motivated to try to pull themselves out of a sea of troubles or driven by frustration to destructive or self-destructive behaviour.

To me a strategy for losers is a strategy that tries to find a way for these groups out of this trapping net of problems. This will only be possible to the extent that last social groups begin to develop the knowledge and abilities to develop their own social, economic and environmental projects and systems of mutual aid. This seems a very ambitious project, but I will argue that this is not as unrealistic as it might seem at first sight – even if much work will be needed to find the best ways of catalysing and supporting the process.

Rethinking what is meant by power and empowerment

Power in human society is not merely taking decisions, it is using energy – whether human energy or physical energy – for a purpose. This involves making and seeing through initiatives. Powerful people and institutions do not just 'take decisions'; they define their own purposes and then plan, design, implement, and monitor projects, exercises and programmes which are suitable to their purposes and their interests. Only when a group or individual develops and oversees the whole of a change process in pursuit of its self-defined purposes can it guarantee that it will be the beneficiary. At the moment we have human and welfare services where the beneficiaries are the workers and the managers rather than the consumers. It is the dissatisfaction with this that has led to the explosive growth of various user and advocacy movements over the last few years. But this movement has had too limited an impact and I believe we must reformulate, or become much clearer about what we mean by 'empowerment' if those groups which I have described as 'last' groups are to define their own purposes and plan their own projects.

A broad conception of empowerment goes beyond just having a voice in a public sector service (like the mental health service). To me it means a situation in which disadvantaged groups or individuals begin to define purposes for themselves and then plan, design, implement and monitor a change process. A catalyst which widens people's horizons about what is possible may be necessary to start the process going. People then start by defining new purposes and new agendas, and then begin to pursue them.

The usual way of thinking about empowerment is that it involves consultation and participation in the decision making and planning of already existing institutions. But these processes are usually attempts to enrol people to legitimise the priorities and agendas of the power centres, or at best to modify their agendas. Consultation and participation can only contribute to empowerment when they advance the agendas and projects of powerless people into the institutions of power. Before getting involved with the health and social services or any other institution of power the crucial question for users to ask is whether it will repay the expenditure of energy and effort in the pursuit of purposes defined by users themselves.

Other meanings of the word empowerment

The idea of empowerment has become very fashionable over the last few years but in the most part it means something rather different from what I have described here. I first came across the term when I was working with others to develop the psychiatric services users' movement in the late 1980s. At that time it meant, for those of us who had used psychiatric services, and for a wider circle in the disability movement, the right to have our voices heard in those health and social services which were supposed to be there to help us. We started a user movement because our experience was that our assumed incompetence was highly magnified and we were devalued as people. While in some places things are marginally better, this is still the experience of many who receive psychiatric services. We were not being listened to, or we were being condescended to, by people who always seemed to assume that they knew better but who rarely did.

As the user movement developed, perhaps partly because it did, empowerment has become a more and more popular term. During the 1980s, at the same time as the user movement was starting to develop, the Tory government were introducing their changes to the health and other public services. Hitherto it had been assumed that the public sector would run effectively if it was merely put in the hands of the great, the good and the wise, and people who had had a professional training. In other words all would be well if controlled by a well-meaning bureaucracy. However, it was difficult to control government expenditure in this way and concern was growing at the cost of welfare services. As Britain declined in the world economy the welfare state seemed to become a bit of a luxury. Napoleon had said England was a nation of shopkeepers and a shopkeeper's daughter started asking if the welfare state was really giving value for money.

New ways were sought to make the public services 'more efficient'. The Thatcher government, convinced that everything must be organised like a profit-making corporation to correspond to their idea of rationality, looked at the public sector in a wholly new way. In the new conventional wisdom people's right to public services were no longer the entitlement of citizens to a guaranteed minimal welfare provision but the demand of customers to measurable and costable packages of services on sale in a context that had to be competitive to be efficient.

Meanwhile even though studies were showing that there was throughout Europe a phenomenon which became called 'the new poverty'; even though policy documents talked about growing problems of a 'dual society' and 'social exclusion'; even though the number of beggars and homeless people on the street was increasing and long-term unemployment and social decomposition was on the up and up; even though the mental health services have continued to operate on the principle of 'let them eat tranquillisers'; even though in increasing areas of our cities drug addiction, criminality and environmental degradation were reaching dangerous levels, in spite of all these circumstances, those of us who were using mental health and other public services could hardly complain because we were being 'empowered' to have a voice as customers in the new welfare market.

Indeed for those of us confident and articulate enough to get involved we have even been given new opportunities to take advantage of our status as 'professional users'. I have been in employment since 1987 as a user development worker. People like myself have had our involvement eagerly sought by a new breed of quality control managers and planners who had to consult the consumers to be in tune with the times. Through their efforts a charter and a mission statement whose wording we have been consulted over has appeared on every wall. Such statements are always couched in such general terminology that they don't tie the services down to anything definite at all. They cannot be considered to be a means through which we have been empowered.

Empowerment must resolve the interlocking problems faced by powerless people

I suggest that the changes which have taken place in the way in which services are organised and managed have done little genuinely to empower people. On a day-to-day basis most of the mental health services still function much as they ever did. The issues raised are the same as ever. Although some of us developed critiques of the medical model and wrote about the need for new approaches, stressing talking treatments and a need for new kinds of services, we have been mostly ignored. Indeed, going beyond this, it is only too evident that the appalling social, economic and environmental conditions in which many users live have got worse. Problems relating to benefits, jobs and accommodation are more difficult. These set the context in which people's personal relations and emotional lives take place, in which mental and physical health problems are caused, or in which people must try to recover from them.

This is not to deny that when the user movement in psychiatry got going, something significant changed. For many people the chance to meet other users and to organise together has been a marvellous step forward. In a few cases it has quite transformed people's lives, brought back confidence in their own abilities and provided opportunities for a real development of their skills. There has been for many of us a real learning process and the development of different ways of thinking about our problems, as well as the search for different ways of solving them. But we have only just got going and I feel we need to make radical rethinks about what genuine empowerment would look like because if what we have now is empowerment, then it is not good enough.

Key elements in a strategy for losers

I will summarise what I see as being the key aspects of a strategy for losers which responds to these interlocking problems and then discuss each idea in more detail.

First, it would be an illusion to believe that severely disempowered people trapped in an interlocking set of problems are completely spontaneously going to set about developing self-help initiatives to improve their social, economic and environmental conditions. Some catalysing processes and support systems are necessary. However, these must not take over and direct the process. They must genuinely work alongside and support an empowerment process that becomes more and more self-sufficient.

Second, the idea of projects generated by powerless people seems to lack credibility if we think of, for example, trying to generate employment by building factories to employ people making aerospace equipment to be sold on a competitive world market. A strategy for losers is about mobilising local unemployed labour and resources to meet local needs as identified by local and poor people. Since the needs that impoverished people have are basic, we are talking about food, shelter, affordable warmth and childcare. This means that instead of thinking of work as something that needs to take place in a factory owned by a multinational operating for a distant market it is more helpful to think of the work that is needed as being neighbourhood and home based.

Third, the environmental crisis is compelling a rethink about how essential needs shall be met to reduce the need for energy-guzzling technologies in vast power and transport networks. The underlying theme for ecological restructuring of the economy implies a move to greater local self-sufficiency for essential needs. And this need for ecological restructuring matches nicely the need to redevelop the homes and neighbourhoods where social deprivation prevails.

Fourth, people immediately ask where the money would come from for such a process. Solving the problem of how resources are mobilised does indeed have to be an integral part of a strategy for losers. But the main problem is not an absence of resources in most areas of poverty – there is commonly much unemployed labour; frequently there are empty or under-utilised buildings or equipment. The real problem is an absence of ways of mobilising these resources as well as the absence of an alternative vision of what they are mobilised for. A number of approaches have been tried in community economic development strategies around the world. Part of the solution lies in finding new, non-monetary means of mobilising resources – like the sophisticated labour and skills exchange system called LETS schemes (see below). Another approach is social banking where wealthy people who are socially responsible are put in touch with positive projects to agree loans and assistance on favourable terms. Even more ambitious, if the political pre-conditions are right, is the idea of local currencies.

In summary, a strategy for losers is an empowerment strategy for last social groups that helps them use their own unemployed labour to solve local economic, social, health and environmental problems in one process – thereby playing a leading role in the economy and society.

Ways to get started – means to catalyse the process

Ways have to be found to help catalyse this process. Means have to be found that will widen people's horizons about what is possible and what they are capable of, support mechanisms have to be set up that really do *support* – without taking over and directing. Professional people and managers who are used to planning project development where there is money which can be used to employ people often totally underestimate the difficulty of doing things without cash and with voluntary labour. That means that although we want to develop things ambitiously in respect of long-term aims, our first steps must be very small-scale and easily achievable.

When an organisation can pay people to do things it can make reasonably accurate estimates of what its employees can achieve and so set up schedules for the course of development. One cannot do this in new projects, run only by people acting as volunteers. At the start, when people come together, they may not know each other. They do not know enough to know what they can expect from each other. Volunteers cannot be depended on. They may wish to stay involved but get blown off course by welfare benefits problems and the need to look for work. They can become involved but become demoralised because what they are involved in cannot quickly enough deliver them the benefits that they want from their voluntary activity.

Keeping all the people involved, because it takes time to achieve an organisation's aims, becomes a major task in its own right. At the start all the roles that would be shared between many different specialists in a larger organisation fall to a very small number of overburdened individuals who are rarely capable of doing absolutely everything perfectly. The sheer variety of new tasks can make it very difficult to plan clear workloads – especially when people are feeling their way in new roles. All those arrangements which enable workers in large organisations to have an uncluttered, undistracted mind, are lacking – a reception that can hold casual callers at bay; a secretary and administrator to do the filing; a place to do the typing which is not also the coffee bar where one is being continually interrupted for irrelevant chats; an office where putting up new shelving or getting a new filing cabinet is yet another task for the same worker who struggles to work there without even a proper desk (at double the time he or she is actually paid for).

Many small projects are funded through grant aid, but grant aid is always available only for practice – never for administration, though the economies of scale in small starting projects would make funding administration a huge percentage in relation to project costs. Project workers may therefore end up doing their own administration; their own clerical work and typing; their own bookkeeping and accounts; their own marketing strategy, development strategy, public relations and recruitment (and recruitment is very different when one is not yet a channel for people pressured to attend through official referral systems). They may struggle with assessments of how far they can delegate these things to volunteers and, if they find they have made the wrong judgement, several weeks later decide they are going to have to do themselves what they thought they had delegated. (Later they may find that they have upset the person whose delegated role has been taken back from them in circumstances that there is not sufficient time to clarify, leaving bad feelings all round.)

Arranging things in the domestic economy at first

Nevertheless, if we start small enough we can get started. Many of the formidable problems of getting things going are solved by arranging things as if they were domestic arrangements between friends as opposed to business arrangements. This has certainly been the experience of my project, 'Ecoworks', which has developed from within the mental health user movement to put into practice many of the ideas discussed here. Much of the work is house- and neighbourhood-orientated and an important feature of a strategy for losers would be an emphasis on work done *outside* the formal economy. Although there does also need to be a strategy for building up more formal arrangements.

The domestic economy (by which I mean informal household-based work) and informal work exchange, if it was given a market valuation, would represent about 60% of British Gross National Product. If home-based activities were paid more in the market it would be much higher. Finnish studies (Pulliainen and Pietila, 1983) show that the domestic economy totals 7 billion hours per year against 6 billion in the formal economy (public and private sectors). It is important to recognise, therefore, that when we add together all those activities which together create human well-being they happen as much, indeed more, outside paid work. The original Greek word from which the words 'economics' and 'ecology' were derived was '*oikos*' meaning 'home'. We need a strategy based on moving back to an integration of the meanings.

Mobilising local unused labour for basic local needs – and simultaneously restructuring the economy for ecological arrangements

An ecological vision centred on restructuring homes and neighbourhoods provides a good focus in a strategy for losers. Ecological restructuring takes its starting point in the home and neighbourhood rather than the workplace (and business). Restructuring production arrangements so that ecological problems are prevented from arising in the first place focuses on housing and neighbourhoods as the key place for change. The following are also best organised in neighbourhood strategies: household insulation; solar heating and voltaic technologies; urban agriculture projects based on forest gardening and permaculture; the separation, composting or reuse of wastes; drink water saving measures, rainwater use, grey water recycling and black water disposal.

Centred on homes and neighbourhoods these changes could be the basis for the redevelopment of areas of decay and relate closely to the need of community care strategies to focus on recreating homes and communities. These changes would require the sorts of skills and labour that is available as unemployed labour in those areas. It would be a small-scale local economics manageable by the entrepreneurial capacities of local people. An ecological vision centred on neighbourhood restructuring would directly affect not only urban ecology but would also improve income (reducing fuel bills, water bills, repair bills etc), improve health through improved physical surroundings, and boost community morale. It would occur in those locations with which disempowered sections of populations are most familiar and, therefore, where they would be most confident in taking and maintaining the initiative – in their own homes and neighbourhoods. It is a strategy that would put women in the driving seat because they would be, quite literally, on home ground. It would also relate directly to the needs of disabled people (for whom building and neighbourhood design are key issues of accessibility and mobility). It would directly connect into issues of community safety – the layout of streets and houses is very important to factors affecting whether crimes take place or not.

The psycho-social dynamics of community development

The importance of collective projects lies in more than merely providing alternative sources of cheap and healthy food, or affordable warmth, or safer streets. Collective initiatives are important to people's emotional health. Community psychologists have found it helps to bring people together to identify what problems they share, and then to try to find collective solutions (Davey, 1994, 1997). Ending isolation and building assertiveness and self-confidence, empowering people, is essential to their psychological well-being. It is this process in all its parts, the package that interweaves ecological renovation of houses and neighbourhoods with community regeneration, that is important. Redevelopment will only be attractive enough if the bigger package rebuilds community support structures, rebuilds community life and people's relationships with each other. Interweaving a popular cultural and artistic component, to make the process enjoyable, is also important. So too is the involvement of children, to the extent that is possible, within their own, self-directed, projects.

There are a host of ways in which redevelopment centred on environmental themes could improve people's relationships and quality of life. Controlling road traffic, for example, would increase welfare in many poor districts. Heavy traffic outside the front door destroys neighbourliness and has been shown to reduce the number of friends people have. English studies have shown dramatic falls in the extent to which children can play and roam outside their houses unsupervised by parents leading to serious deterioration in their emotional and physical development (Hillman, 1993).

Organisational vehicles for change – the Atlantis model in Berlin

These ideas have been implemented in Berlin in a number of projects promoting local economic development from the community and neighbourhood level. The community economic self-help and local economic development movement has held two international conferences and its ideas are become increasingly widely known. One of the Berlin projects which was a participant in both international conferences is called Atlantis. Atlantis evolved out of a social work rehabilitation agency for young people who have had mental health problems. It takes young people and trains them in environment technologies. When I first visited Atlantis it trained or employed 300 people in wind energy, solar energy, measures to improve the energy efficiency of buildings and projects to green neighbourhoods. I decided that, as a development worker, newly starting with the Nottingham Advocacy Group, I would like to develop something similar in

Nottingham to put users at the head of an economic process which is liable to run for the next 30 or so years.

The Ecoworks model in Nottingham

Our project, called 'Ecoworks'[2], has been created out of an alliance between people in the mental health user movement and green professionals to be a Nottingham Atlantis. We have had to adapt our vision to our local resources and conditions but after three years we had a number of small projects funded by joint finance, social services grant aid and Nottinghamshire County Council green grant initiative. Subsequently we obtained National Lottery funding and have been able to employ our first full-time worker and move to our own office.

We still have contacts with Atlantis and a number of German projects and hope to build on them. Since we started Ecoworks, Atlantis has proved the potential of the new technologies and grown to 450 trainees and employees. It is the largest employer in the Kreuzberg district of Berlin. Through our contacts with it and other German projects, for example the Bauhaus Dessau, we have become recognised as experts on green economic questions in Nottingham and Nottinghamshire and have been invited to participate in a variety of international conferences. We hope to capitalise on this soon with bids into Europe.

Funding and means to mobilise resources

At the very start of the process we got going through a social services grant to my development project, followed by mental health joint finance. Later we hope that European money can begin to build up the scale of what we can do. In the meantime other means of mobilising local resources need to be looked at. Elsewhere in Nottingham some colleagues, also based at the Nottingham Advocacy Group, are hoping to develop a project adapting the LETS scheme that I mentioned earlier.

People who join LETS can do jobs for other people in the scheme at an agreed price, but no money need actually change hands. Each person joining the scheme gives details of their wants and jobs that they are prepared to do. A central administration compiles a list of the wants and skills on offer. Through this list people contact each other. When they either do work or receive work in the system they let the central administration know how much it was valued at and this figure is recorded. The amount registered after each transaction entitles the service provider to get work or goods to that value from someone else in the system. Those who received a service or good are obliged in a reasonable period of time to do a roughly equivalent amount of work for someone else in the system.

LETS systems are a way of mobilising resources without money – they are needed because poor people often have wants and skills but no money. There is little money in poor areas. Money tends to drain away into centres of power and economic activity so new means have to be found to mobilise unemployed resources. The question is how, and for what purpose, these resources can be mobilised. There are cases in the economic history of this century which show us that local communities that have found local means to mobilise local resources – like sophisticated barter trading systems, or even local currencies – have had dramatic success in reducing local unemployment. This was the experience in the inter-war experiment at Worgl in Austria.

A concluding summary

To summarise – a strategy for losers is about disempowered sections of society developing projects that use their own resources to meet their essential needs in their local environments. It is about developing the capacity to provide essential needs in new ways and simultaneously installing the 'soft energy', organic technologies of the future. If the political will were there, matching and supportive policies would encourage this development. Social, health, environmental and economic policy could be creatively combined to enable disadvantaged people to develop an economic role as they improved their own environment.

Notes

[1] The themes discussed in this chapter are developed in a forthcoming book entitled *Strategien gegen Ausgrenzung* (Strategies against exclusion) to be published by Manx Verlag Schulbuch, Vienna.

[2] Ecoworks (Nottingham) Ltd, 9a Forest Road East, Nottingham NG1 4HJ, UK Tel +44 (0)115 948 4111.

References

Davey, B. (1994) 'Madness and its causative contexts', *International Journal of Psychology and Psychotherapy*, vol 12, no 2, pp 113-32.

Davey, B. (1997) 'Meaning, madness and recovery', *Clinical Psychology Forum*, vol 103, May, p 19.

Hillman, M. (ed) (1993) *Children, transport and quality of life*, London: Policy Studies Institute.

Pulliainen, K. and Pietila, H. (1983) 'Revival of non monetary economy makes economic growth unnecessary', *IDFD*, Dossier 77.

An idea for action

The idea of setting up user forums came from three directions: from managers, clinical staff and users. The Trust wanted to encourage users to respond to an important health authority consultation document on the siting of inpatient services. We discovered that there was no structured way of asking service users what they thought about these or any other proposals. Senior managers of the Trust believed that service users had both a right to a voice in decision making and an expertise on which the Trust should draw. They asked me to explore possible ways of finding out from users how services could be improved and what needed to be done to make the Trust more responsive to their needs. Developing user forums was one way for managers and staff to find out users' views which seemed to offer possibilities for the Trust.

Shortly after I was approached by senior managers of the Trust, one or two staff in the mental health service asked my advice about the idea of a Patients' Council, a formal user-led forum, where users from different wards could get together to discuss the service. One difficulty with this scheme was that people were inpatients for a brief spell, and were only in hospital at a point when their particular problems became overwhelming. How could we make sure that there was some continuity from one meeting to the next and that the Councils did not fall away after a short period, leaving everyone disillusioned? Nevertheless, raising the idea of a Council suggested that staff were looking for ways to listen to users.

Around this time, the Trust hosted a 'Stakeholder Conference' for groups and individuals with a stake in mental health services, including user groups, voluntary groups, purchasers, providers, social services and any other interested parties. In a workshop I attended, users and managers shared ideas for future user involvement in services. During this workshop it transpired that social services day centres had established user groups, and users involved in these volunteered to help staff in health services to learn from their experience. This appeared to provide a focus for my proposed action research and an opportunity for Trust staff to engage in development work.

Learning from the literature

The first step for me was to undertake a literature search so I could learn from previous research and practice. I was particularly interested to find out what had been done in other parts of the country both to involve users in mental health services and to set up user forums. I became interested by the debate on the differences and links between consumer involvement and citizen involvement. The literature suggests that the focus of consumerism is on making services responsive to the individual, and on aggregating those individual choices to influence the nature and range of services provided (Winkler, 1987; Potter, 1988; Ong, 1993). Citizenship, on the other hand, implies involvement in decision making: for individuals in their own care and treatment, for user groups and interest groups in influencing services, and for the wider public through representative and possibly direct democracy (Klein, 1984; Hambleton, 1988; Croft and Beresford, 1992; Barnes and Wistow, 1993). Another theme that I went on to read around was that of empowerment, and different ways of thinking about power. This enabled me to reflect on how any action would need to take into account the concerns of staff about losing their power (Higgins, 1993; Glenister, 1994). I read about the different ways that users had become involved in trying to change services, and the things that they said about what was important to them, such as having a user-only group (Chamberlin, 1987; Robson, 1987; Campbell, 1990), and the importance of action as well as discussion (Hutchinson et al, 1990; Barnes and Wistow, 1994a, 1994b). It seemed the right time for me to move on from thinking to action.

First thoughts

The plan of action had three stages. First, I would find an existing staff team that wanted to set up a user forum, and take up the offer of user volunteers from the day centres to help support the forum. In this way the forum would be user-led rather than staff-led, but external user input would provide some continuity in the context of the rapidly changing patient population of the particular service. Second, patients and user volunteers would hold some user-only meetings, inform the staff of users' concerns and the staff would discuss and act on the concerns raised. Finally, the staff, patients and user volunteers together would evaluate the success or failure of the user forums, considering what had contributed to or hindered their success.

What actually happened

Preparing the staff

I wrote to the managers of the various nursing teams in the mental health directorate, asking if I could talk to them about user involvement, and particularly about setting up a forum as part of a research project. Over the period of the project, I talked to five inpatient and two day service managers, and three community teams. As each meeting took place, what I learnt strengthened the initial impression that the more immediate need was not my idea of a user forum, but increasing staff awareness of what user involvement might mean and helping teams to think about how to extend it.

One theme that I had picked out from the literature as relevant was the need to prepare staff to involve users (Beeforth et al, 1990; Hutchinson et al, 1990; Higgins, 1993). Several authors suggest that staff may be reluctant to share power with service users (Berry, 1988; Beeforth et al, 1990; Glenister, 1994). The preparation needed, it is implied, is helping staff to come to terms with the change in power relationships, and to view it positively. However, rather than discovering reservations about the abilities of users, or anxieties about the potential loss of control, I found that staff appeared to be genuinely interested in involving users. They told me that they were interested in doing more, but were not sure what to do. This was combined with some complacency about current practice, and certainly a narrow focus on particular elements of involvement, such as user satisfaction surveys or staff-led 'community meetings'.

Despite the assertion that users already had available a variety of means to put forward their views (through formal complaints procedures, through an informal grumble and suggestion scheme and through speaking to individual staff), the teams did not set aside any time for examining what information they had from these sources about improving the service. Individual problems might be resolved, but there was no way of looking at all of the information and drawing out patterns, picking up on good ideas, or acting on what service users said collectively. This had implications for setting up a user forum, because the teams had no existing process to discuss and act on what the users were already telling them. I felt it was essential to the success of a forum that they developed such a process and the determination to act on it (Hutchinson et al, 1990; Barnes and Wistow, 1994b, 1994c).

Having looked at the idea of user forums with staff and having reflected on what I had learnt, I concluded that the key issue seemed to be helping teams both to think more about user involvement in their area, and to identify the best way forward in their circumstances. This needed to include ways of acting on what they learnt from users.

Finding user volunteers

There was more of a problem in finding user volunteers than I had anticipated at the start of the project. I wrote to the two social service day centres whose users had said they would help, addressing the letter to 'the users'. The staff of one centre wrote back to suggest I attend a centre meeting and that I ring them (the staff) to confirm I could attend. As I had addressed the letter to the users of the centre, it began to emerge that user involvement might not be quite as well developed as had been suggested at the Stakeholder Conference. The second centre did not reply formally, so I asked some of the users I had come to know about their involvement within the centre. A group of users there were taking the lead in an innovative project to use a centre building as an evening and weekend social centre. Despite this, there were no user-only meetings that advised on or contributed to the management of the centres. This was mirrored by the other centre when I took up their invitation to visit. In both centres users and staff had joint meetings at which centre business was discussed. Most of the literature written by users that I was reading recommended meeting without staff present (Chamberlin, 1987; Robson, 1987; Campbell, 1990). This allows users to feel free to say what they want. It did not appear that such a model was currently being used in the city. The network that I thought I had, of user volunteers with experience in leading user forums, did not exist.

This set me thinking about what might be needed to support users in taking the idea forward. I was influenced by three things: a visit to users in Nottingham, a seminar paper given by a user of mental health services, Brian Davey (see Brian Davey's contribution in this book, pp 37-49), and a series of discussions with the local Sheffield Mental Health Forum. In Nottingham I talked to a service user who had been involved in developing Patients' Councils and self-advocacy there. He explained that the initial work on Patients' Councils was undertaken by a group of users who identified themselves as volunteers, and supported each other. The main focus of their early work was on improving the service, and they worked with allies in health and social services.

A week later I went to a seminar in the 'Alliances and Participation in Empowerment' series where Davey, a user from Nottingham, presented a paper about his experiences. He had initially been involved as a volunteer in trying to change services but had become disillusioned and had moved on to working with others on sustainable community development. Davey talked about the issue of agendas. He said:

> Consultation and participation are the usual ways that power centres think of involving other people – but these are usually attempts to enrol others in support of the priorities and agendas of the power centres themselves, in support of their own initiatives.

The Mental Health Forum in Sheffield was set up to work for change in the local mental health field. It has attracted workers and users from both the voluntary sector and statutory services, and has taken different forms over the years. In the 12 months prior to this study, there had been an increasing focus on users taking more of a lead in the Forum, and in thinking about what they wanted to do. The user members of the Forum identified the need for users to be trained and supported to do this (cf Beeforth et al, 1990; Hutchinson et al, 1990). I realised that there was a tension developing for me between my agenda, which was to recruit users to help staff within the Trust improve services, and the users' need to develop their own agenda. As I thought more about this I realised that I had to put the user agenda first (Campbell, 1990; Lindow, 1994).

The next steps

In the light of this I felt the most important thing was for the Trust to give support to users in developing their agenda. Local users participating in the Mental Health Forum were thus encouraged in their desire to establish an autonomous user group. The group currently meets in a Trust building, providing them with an address and the use of a phone, though it is hoping to move out to an office shortly. The users have taken over the running of the local Mental Health Forum, and have started a magazine. They are still discussing how they want to work to bring about changes in the services they use, and I have had some meetings with them to discuss how we can work together. There has been some discussion about peer advocacy and about the group working with users of inpatient services to improve the services they get. There are no firm plans to put this into action, because the user group wants to set the pace.

At a wider level, work has gone on to prepare the ground for more user involvement. One of the day centres has set up a forum, supported by an ex-user. The staff have found this challenging, but enjoyable, and have made changes to their practice, such as wearing name badges, and making sure that users have time with their keyworkers regularly.

Within the Trust as a whole, I used the information from talking to users, and from the literature, to develop a framework to help teams within the Trust to think about user involvement. This framework has been incorporated into the Trust's *Strategy for community participation and user involvement*. I have used the framework with a number of teams to help them identify how to increase the involvement of service users. The framework is based on two concepts from the literature on user involvement.

The first is about the focus or level of involvement. It takes into account concepts from consumerism and citizenship. In describing how consumerism can be applied in mental health practice, Renshaw (1987) suggests four levels of involvement: individual service plans; asking views of groups at the level of the service unit; consumer representatives contributing to planning; and education and awareness for the general public. Similar but expanded levels of involvement of the user and citizen are described in Barnes and Wistow (1992), widening from the individual, to groups, to management and planning of services, to resource management and planning, to policy making in an agency, to inter-agency work and thence to national involvement. The importance of focusing involvement at a number of levels is stressed by several authors (Beeforth et al, 1990; Hutchinson et al, 1990; Barnes and Wistow, 1992; Philpot, 1994).

The second concept is the idea of an increasing amount, or ladder, of participation, which has been widely used in considering user involvement (Arnstein, 1969; Smith, 1987; Quayoom, 1990; NHSTD, 1993; Philpot, 1994). Whatever the level or focus of involvement, in individual care planning up to national level, it is important to be clear and honest about how much power the user has to influence decision making. The remainder of this paper will describe the user involvement framework and the way in which I used it with staff teams in the Trust.

A user involvement framework

Reproduced below is the paper setting out the details of the approach which I produced for the Trust.

A framework for thinking about user involvement

There is a lot of interest in involving the people who use our services in what we do as a Trust. However, though we want to do this, there is a lot of uncertainty about how to go about it. This sets out a way of thinking about what we can do to involve people. You can use the ideas in here to identify what you are doing already, and to plan what you might want to do next.

Asking what? and who?
We want to find a way of thinking about involving people in everything we do, not just in unimportant things around the edges. The first key questions we need to ask ourselves are:

- what exactly is it that we want to involve people in?
- who, then, do we want to involve?
- who should be doing this?

What?
To do a really good job in involving people, we want to involve them in:

- their own treatment and care;
- contributing to the management and decision making of the services they use regularly;
- changing and improving services;
- developing and shaping future services.

Who to involve in what?
One way of thinking about who we should involve is to start with what concerns people:

- most importantly, having some control over what happens to them as individuals;
- secondly, helping improve the service they are using, in common with others;
- having a say in how services are developed; this is particularly true for those who will need services over a long time and have an interest or stake in the future of that service;
- the public have an interest in health services, both as potential users and taxpayers.

This widening focus of potential involvement can be depicted as follows:

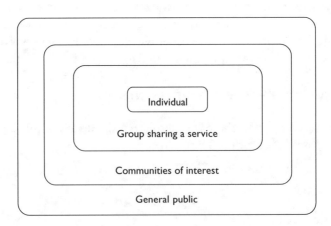

Individual

Group sharing a service

Communities of interest

General public

We are therefore talking about involving:

Individual users (including informal carers where appropriate)
We need to remember that this means each person using the Trust's services. We need to involve them so they have a say in their own treatment. The people who can make this happen are clinical staff, and they need to be supported by their management teams.

Groups of people sharing a particular service
By this we mean people who have a common interest because they are all current users of the same part of a service. They might attend the same clinic, be an inpatient on the same ward or be clients of a community health team. We might want to invite them to contribute to the decision making in their service, and they are likely to have ideas about how to improve it. There need to be clearly identified ways for encouraging contributions and ideas. This is the particular concern of the managers of a service. Using such systems effectively is the concern of teams providing a service.

Communities of interest
A community of interest, in this context, means people who have a shared interest in a particular service because they have used it, are using it or might need to use it in the future. Examples might be users of mental health services, or carers of people with learning disabilities. It might also be people with specific needs and concerns such as black and minority ethnic communities. These communities of interest have ideas about how services should change and develop, and we should be treating their expertise as a valuable resource. As all health and social service purchasers and providers need to tap into this resource, it is a waste of everyone's time not to do this jointly. In the Trust therefore, Clinical Advisory Groups should be examining ways of multi-agency working to involve these communities, and management teams should be identifying and strengthening their links with them.

General public
The public have a right to comment on and influence health service planning. To do this, they need to be aware of the relevant issues. Involving the public is mainly the responsibility of the health purchasers, but is also a concern of senior managers and practitioners in the Trust.

A way of summarising this is:

Who should we involve?	**Individual users/carers**	**Groups sharing same service**	**Communities of interest**	**General public**
In what should we involve them?	Taking as much control as possible of their treatment and care	Contributing to the decision making in the service they are using. Improving services	Improving services. Developing new ideas and new services	A greater understanding of health issues. Influencing planning and priorities
Who should be doing this?	Clinical staff, supported by their management team	Clinical and management teams responsible for a service	Management teams. Planning groups, usually jointly with purchasers and other providers	Mainly purchasers. Senior managers and clinical staff

Asking how much?

We know that we have to be practical and that at some times it is easier to involve people than at others. Having decided what we want to involve people in, and who we should involve, we need to ask a second important question:

- How much do we want, or are we able, to involve people? How much of our power can we share with service users?

A common tool for thinking about this is to use a 'ladder' of increasing involvement. We can use this to think of different ways of involving people. A summary of how the 'ladder' idea can be used is as follows:

Power shared	How much can/ does the Trust want to involve people?	What does this mean?
Least power	**Give information**	Letting people know what is happening. Giving people enough information to enable them to make informed choice.
	Gather ideas/ consult	Using people's expertise as service users to get new ideas about how to do things. Asking people what they think about plans and proposals.
	Work together	Working with users who want to help the Trust change, in working parties, project groups, through evaluation, audit and through users as trainers.
Most power	**Supporting user-led initiatives**	Helping user groups through providing training, use of Trust premises, business planning advice, and acting as champions inside Trust systems.

Moving from the minimum to the maximum way of sharing power, we can explore the implications of this in more detail.

Giving information

This means making sure we tell people what is happening. It also means giving people enough information so they can decide what they want to happen.

To make this work we need:
- to find out from users what they want to know, as well as thinking about what we have to tell them;
- to have suitable material
    - jargon-free
    - in different languages, including signing and symbols
    - in different media, such as written, audiotapes and videos;
- to be clear about who needs to receive information;
- to be clear about who is responsible for giving information.

Gathering ideas and consulting

At its worst, a consultation exercise can be undertaken when there is little scope for change, raising expectations that cannot be met. This is often user, carer and voluntary groups' past experience. Consultation by the Trust should mean using people's expertise as service users to get new ideas about how to do things. It should also mean asking them what they think about our ideas, plans and proposals.

To make this work we need
- to identify the ways we gather new ideas, through
  surveys
  focus groups
  supporting regular meetings of our users/carers
  developing links with user/carer/voluntary groups, and going out to listen to them;
- to set aside a regular time to discuss what we have learnt, in clinical and management team meetings;
- to decide who makes sure something is done about good ideas;
- to identify the way we tell users what is being done about their ideas;
- to be clear about who we should consult with on our new ideas (the Trust has an up-to-date database list of groups in the Quality Department office.)

Working together
The Trust need to draw on users' expertise to work up the detail of ideas and proposals. We can do this by asking users to help us on working groups, or by joining our regular meetings. Users may also want to be involved in decision making, in evaluating or auditing services, or in training staff.

To make this work we need
- to identify who are the people, and groups, who are willing to help us. We need to think carefully about what the advantages and disadvantages are for both sides in any proposal to work together. Is it worth the user's time and energy?
- to make sure that anyone who is willing to help us gets the information they need. We need to remember they will need information about the context of the work, as well as just the task in hand.
- to hold meetings at a time and place that is suitable for users. Many users and carers will find it difficult to make it to a meeting that starts at 9 am, or that has no disabled access or is not on a bus route.
- to make sure that people do not have to pay for getting involved. Transport and carer costs will need to be met.

Supporting user initiatives and agendas
People may be willing and able to provide a particular service for themselves. This might range from setting up a self-help group, to running a drop-in centre. It may be that users can act as paid consultants, for example, in giving advice on access, or in running training for us. We need to remember that involvement is not just about what we want to discuss, but about issues on which users want to focus.

The Trust can help user groups in a variety of ways:
- providing training
- allowing use of Trust premises
- business planning advice
- acting as champions inside statutory organisations.
- employing user consultants in appropriate circumstances.

Making this into a framework
Having thought about some of these questions, we can put them together to form a grid. The grid can then be used, as a whole or by column, to identify what your team does already to involve people:

It is mainly the responsibility of: >	clinicians and their managers	clinical teams and directorates	planning groups, directorates	purchaser, managers
To involve >	**Individual users/ carers (in planning their treatment)**	**Groups sharing same service (in managing and improving services)**	**Communities of interest (in improving and developing service)**	**General public**
By				
Giving information				
Gathering ideas/ consulting				●
Working together				
Supporting user initiatives and agendas				

Each team will need to decide which aspects (columns) are most relevant to themselves. For each box in the grid or column teams might want ask themselves:

- what do we do already?
- what *could* we do to improve involvement? Eg:

	Individual users/carers (in planning their treatment)
Giving information	What do we do already to give relevant information? What *could* we do to increase the information users have?

Here are some of the questions your team might want to ask about each aspect:

	Individual users/carers
Giving information	Have you asked users what information they want? Have you got information packs about all the treatments (including drugs) you offer? Have you checked that there is no jargon? Is it available in different languages? Is it on tape or video? How do you make sure everyone gets the information? Is it clear who is responsible for providing it to the user/carer?
Gathering ideas and consulting	How do you agree with users and carers what are the main problems to be tackled in treatment? Who describes the problem and who writes it down?
Working together	Who keeps the information/treatment plan? How do you involve people in multi-disciplinary planning, recognising the difficulty for users in speaking out in a roomful of professionals? Do you use advocates?
Supporting user initiatives	How do you let people know about self-help groups? Do you provide users with self-help and educational material?

	Groups sharing same service
Giving information	Have you got information about the services you provide, that users have helped to produce? Have you checked that there is no jargon? Is this available in different languages? Is it on tape or video? How do you make sure everyone gets the information? When do they get it?
Gathering ideas and consulting	How do you ask people what they think? Do you set aside a regular time to discuss users' ideas? How do you make sure they get translated into action? How do you make sure you tell the users what has been done?
Working together	How often do you involve people in the meetings you have? How do you get users to help you when you do something new, such as produce a new information sheet, change the way a clinic runs, redecorate a building?
Supporting user initiatives and agendas	How do you support self-help groups (with publicity, rooms, liaison)? Do you have a named link with the relevant user-led groups and carer groups? How do you make sure that you discuss the things that users want to raise, as well as involving them in the things that are important to you?
	Communities of interest
Giving information	Who do you need to keep informed about your services? Have you a comprehensive list of groups and individuals? How do you present information to them?
Gathering ideas/ consulting	How do you link into existing forums? How often do you go out to user, carer and local groups? Do you have an identified link person for each group relevant to your area of work ?
Working together	How do you identify those users who are interested in helping you? How do you contact them?
Supporting user initiatives and agendas	What happens when users want to provide a service for themselves? Do you help them or regard them as a business threat? How do you develop an agenda that includes user priorities as well as your own?

Have you identified all the appropriate communities? **Are you working with other statutory organisations towards a joint approach? If not, why not?**

Conclusion
Involving our service users needs to be a dynamic process. It is not possible, nor desirable, to be prescriptive about what each team should be doing. The only thing that we can say is that every team should be doing something, and that they should be changing and adapting what they do to involve people, in the light of what they learn. This grid may help you think about what you and your team can do. If you choose not to use it, that's fine. However, you still have to identify clearly what you are doing, and what you will do next, to involve service users.

Does the framework work?

The framework was widely distributed within the Trust, with the aim of stimulating different teams to identify steps they could take to involve users. I also made presentations to approximately fifteen planning and clinical teams across different clinical areas, selecting the most appropriate aspect of the grid for them to use. On these occasions, clinical teams usually applied the framework in relation to the groups that used their service, planning teams the communities of interest. The process thus included services for children and young people, for older people, for people with learning disabilities, with mental health problems, and community services. Working in pairs, I asked the staff present to identify any action they were already taking to involve people, and to identify at least one further action they could take to increase involvement. The response was variable. Most teams managed to identify some things that they already did, for example provide information leaflets or self-help material; regular reviews of suggestion schemes and user-satisfaction information; regular contact with some of the local or self-help groups. Most of the teams were surprised that they were doing anything at all, as they perceived user involvement to be something completely new, that they needed to learn how to do. The framework helped them to think of it as a process that they had often already begun, and that they could use to identify the next step. Thus if teams were interested in involving users, it could help them think through ways of doing this. Most staff and managers believed it was right that people should have a strong voice in their treatment and the service available. This was balanced by the recognition that treatment also needed to be a partnership with clinical staff. At all the sessions I ran people expressed the desire to deliver a good service, and they recognised that involving users would help them do this. It was, therefore, seen as being mutually beneficial to users and staff.

What the framework cannot do is convince staff who do not want to involve service users to do so. Most of the teams with whom I used the framework had expressed an interest. Some of the teams, however, raised potential obstacles. The most common of these were: their clients were dispersed and it would therefore be difficult to get a common view; their clients would find it difficult to contribute because they were too young, or too disabled by dementia or severe disability; and only the most vocal would have a voice so the involvement would be skewed. Some of these teams used the framework to identify steps they could take to involve people, some remained unconvinced.

The weakness of the framework is that it does not change or challenge staff attitudes to users. If they wish, staff groups can use it to confirm limited user involvement. Unless they go on to discuss their views and plans with their service users, they can be falsely complacent and unaware of a host of issues that users want addressed. However, if it is used as a way of getting a dialogue with users started, it can be very effective. As a result of using the framework, some groups have run day conferences with users, have developed links with local groups, have invited user and carer members on to planning groups. Some teams have reviewed information with users to make it more appropriate. These are small steps in a long process.

Conclusion

The framework was developed as a tool for clinical and planning teams to use to structure their approach to user involvement. It has been most useful for those staff teams who already had an interest in taking some action in this area. While it has given some confidence and ideas to teams who had less focus, it has not made any impact on those teams who were not interested in the idea of increasing user involvement. It has to be seen in the context of helping staff to prepare to engage with users, and is not a substitute for concurrent work with users to help them develop their agenda, and thus to determine how they want to be involved.

Notes

[1] I do not intend here to debate the nature of action research, only to describe, as honestly as I can, my experiences of undertaking such a project.

References

Arnstein, S. (1969) 'A ladder of citizen participation in the USA', *Journal of the American Institute of Planners*, vol 35, no 2, pp 216-24.

Barnes, M. and Wistow, G. (1992) 'Understanding user involvement', in M. Barnes and G. Wistow (eds) *Researching user involvement*, Leeds: Nuffield Institute for Health, University of Leeds, pp 1-15.

Barnes, M. and Wistow, G. (1993) *Gaining influence, gaining support: Working with carers in research and practice*, Leeds: Nuffield Institute for Health, University of Leeds.

Barnes, M. and Wistow, G. (1994a) *User-oriented community care*, Leeds: Nuffield Institute for Health, University of Leeds.

Part Two:

Issues for research and researchers

Introduction to Part Two

At the same time that the 1980s and 1990s were witnessing the self-organisation of user groups, researchers were beginning to question their practices and ways in which they might, albeit unwittingly, reinforce top-down perspectives within welfare services. The more reflective approaches to research advocated by feminists (see Introduction and the contribution by France) were being applied, not least, within policy-related matters (Finch, 1981; Warren, 1990). Researchers who are themselves disabled and/or the users of services have critiqued academic research and the research process as potentially disempowering experiences (Morris, 1991, 1995; Barnes and Mercer, 1996; Thomas, 1997). There is increasing evidence that the views of service users can be solicited through more sensitive research approaches and through enabling people to take ownership of the research process itself, via self- and citizen-advocacy projects and quality assurance systems, for example (Grant, 1997).

An increasing number of the main funding bodies for research now require researchers to show how and to what extent users have been involved in the drawing-up of research proposals and/or subsequent plans for the designs and execution of the research[1]. Armchair researchers can no longer remain closeted within academic institutions, though researchers committed to working with or for users may still feel the pull of mainstream academic tradition and the pressures in universities to produce 'output' targets for Research Assessment Exercise (RAE) ratings. Commentators have also noted how the incorporation of users' needs into various aspects of the research process is driven as much by an emphasis on value for money of public services as concern with quality of life. In many instances, requiring the inclusion of users may be little more than a cosmetic exercise (Rappert, 1997).

Despite shifts in philosophies and funding systems, there is still little commentary on or analysis of the effect of user involvement on research itself. The aim of the second part of the collection is not to offer a definitive 'empowerment' method of carrying out research. Rather, it is to consider different ways of enabling people to participate actively in research and to reflect on issues of collaboration within that process. A key question raised concerns over the ownership of research and the potential to exploit or exclude participants. Indeed, common themes emerging from accounts of researchers' experiences include the need to address issues of power and potential conflicts of interest between researchers, users, service providers and other relevant participants. Adequate resources are necessary to prepare for research projects which secure the involvement of service users. Researchers must be skilled in communicating with users, recognising the impact of generational differences as much as hearing impairment or learning disabilities. Finally, although not a central topic in this collection, the importance of dissemination as an integral part of the research process should also be acknowledged (Rappert, 1997).

Alan France and Nina Biehal provide perspectives on attempting to involve participants in research projects with pre-established briefs. France illustrates the ways in which the structure and demands of collecting data impacted upon efforts to gain access to younger people's experiences of Youth Action Projects. He offers a very open account in which he reveals his own lack of clarity as a researcher about how to devise, implement and put into practice ideals about empowering methods. He shows how, in the context of carrying out large-scale, government-funded, evaluative projects, the pressure to produce answers to specific questions can lead to superficial gestures towards involvement. Highlighting the lack of power that is experienced by young people leaving care both as citizens and as service users, Biehal stresses the importance for researchers of giving attention to their rights. She describes strategies used to enable young people to have a say in her study which include local discussion groups, project groups and individual interviews. A range of issues relating to confidence, confidentiality, training and support are highlighted.

Marian Barnes considers the experience of working on an initiative in which empowerment was the driving force. Indeed, the Fife User Panels Project recruited older people not involved in the panels to interview panel members about their involvement. Barnes describes the process of engaging volunteers in designing and conducting the evaluation, and the subsequent benefits to participants in their increased knowledge of local resources including those of potential value to themselves. However, she also acknowledges the boundaries placed on the development of the volunteers' skills by her doubt in their ability to manage other than a structured approach to interviews, especially within time constraints.

As Lorna Warren shows in the conclusion, there is as great a need for researchers to question 'the system' within which they carry out their activities as there is for those who work within health and social care agencies. Academics are equally eager and arrogant in their assertion of expertise. However, collaboration is not a rational, pre-determined process but one in which goals, needs and the criteria for quality are negotiated. It raises questions about the meaning of relevance, the appropriateness of research methodologies, and the epistemological and political status of knowledge (Rappert, 1997). But, if academics are to make a case for the role of research in forwarding understanding of user involvement, they need to be open to users reflecting on their own academic backyard (Warren, 1998). Not only would this represent a step on the path to empowerment for users, it may well help to increase the effectiveness and empowerment of researchers themselves (Maiteny, 1996). Additional texts which explore research-related issues and the notion of empowerment are listed below.

Brief bibliography

Barnes, M. (1995) 'Partnerships in research: working with groups', in G. Wilson (ed) *Community care: Asking the users*, London: Chapman and Hall, pp 228-41.

Barnes, M. and Wistow, G. (eds) (1992) *Researching user involvement*, Leeds: Nuffield Institute for Health, University of Leeds.

Barnes, M. and Wistow, G. (1995) *Gaining influence, gaining support. Working with carers in research and practice*, Leeds: Nuffield Institute for Health, University of Leeds.

Beresford, P. (1997) *Personal accounts: Involving disabled children in research*, London: The Stationery Office.

Beresford, P. and Harding, T. (eds) (1993) *A challenge to change: Practical experiences of building user-led services*, London: National Institute for Social Work.

Cooper, M. and Sidell, M. (1994) *Lewisham older women's health survey*, London: EdROP The City Lit.

Disability, Handicap and Society (1992) vol 7, no 2, Special Issue: 'Researching disability'.

Moore, M., Beazley, S. and Maelzer, J. (1998) *Researching disability issues*, Buckingham: Open University Press.

Morris, J. (ed) (1996) *Encounters with strangers: Feminism and disability*, London: The Women's Press.

Rioux, M. and Bach, M. (eds) (1994) *Disability is not measles: New research paradigms in disability*, Ontario: Roeher Institute.

Shakespeare, P., Atkinson, D. and French, S. (eds) (1993) *Reflecting on research practice: Issues in health and social welfare*, Buckingham: Open University Press.

Thornton, P. and Tozer, R. (1994) *Involving older people in planning and evaluating community care: A review of initiatives*, York: SPRU, University of York.

Tozer, R. and Thornton, P. (1995) *A meeting of minds: Older people as research advisers*, York: SPRU, University of York.

Ward, L. (1997) *Seen and heard: Involving disabled children and young people in research and development projects*, York: Joseph Rowntree Foundation in association with York Publishing Services Ltd.

Notes

[1] The Department of Health 'Health in Partnership' policy research programme requires researchers submitting bids to demonstrate how they have consulted with users in drawing up their proposals. The DoH has also established a 'Standing Advisory Committee on Consumer Involvement in the NHS R & D Programme'.

The Joseph Rowntree Foundation set out a number of interests that run through their work, regardless of the particular subject area, of which proposers are expected to take account, wherever relevant. First in the list is the importance of service users' perspectives and of involving users in the decisions that affect them. The Foundation declares itself as having "a commitment to exploring ways of ensuring that people central to the research are involved in, and empowered by, the experience" (from the Joseph Rowntree Foundation website at http://www.jrf.org.uk/jrfinfo.html#8). It also expects that all proposals will incorporate race, racism and issues confronting minority ethnic communities. One of the key features of assessment of proposals is whether partnerships with relevant organisations and service users are in place, where these are important.

References

Barnes, C. and Mercer, G. (eds) (1996) *Exploring the divide: Illness and disability*, Leeds: The Disability Press.

Finch, J. (1981) ' "It's great to have someone to talk to": the ethics and politics of interviewing women', in C. Bell and H. Roberts (eds) (1984) *Social researching: Politics, problems, practice*, London: Routledge and Kegan Paul, pp 70-88.

Grant, G. (1997) 'Consulting to involve or consulting to empower?', in P. Ramcharan, G. Roberts, G. Grant, and J. Borland (eds) *Empowerment in everyday life: Learning disability*, London and Bristol: Jessica Kingsley, pp 121-43.

Maiteny, P. (1996) 'Empowering anthropology and the rhetoric of empowerment', *Anthropology in Action*, vol 3, no 1, pp 45-57.

Morris, J. (1991) *Pride against prejudice: Transforming attitudes to disability*, London: The Women's Press.

Morris, J. (1995) 'Creating a space for absent voices: disabled women's experience of receiving assistance with daily living activities', *Feminist Review*, vol 51, Autumn, pp 68-93.

Rappert, B. (1997) 'Users and social science research: policy, problems and possibilities', *Sociological Research Online*, vol 2, no 3. <http://www.socresonline.org.uk/socresonline/2/3/10.html

Thomas, C. (1997) 'The baby and the bathwater: disabled women and motherhood in social context', *Sociology of Health and Illness*, vol 19, no 5, pp 622-43.

Warren, L. (1990) *Doing, being, writing: Research on home care for older people*, Feminist Praxis, monograph number 31.

Warren, L. (1998) 'Considering the culture of community care: anthropological accounts of the experiences of frontline carers, older people and a researcher', in I. Edgar and A. Russell (eds) *The anthropology of welfare*, London: Routledge, pp 183-208.

Exploitation or empowerment? Gaining access to young people's reflections on crime prevention strategies

Alan France

This paper is about empowerment and the research process. It aims to discuss how the structure and demands of collecting data or making discoveries can influence the outcomes of research that aims to be empowering for its participants. By drawing upon experiences from recent research into the effectiveness of youth services in producing crime prevention strategies I will show how a fine line exists between the concepts of exploitation and empowerment and how certain methods of including young people may contradict the good intentions of researchers who aim for empowerment.

The political context of empowerment

Throughout the 1990s, political interest in the concepts of empowerment and participation has generated a growing discourse on the importance of such ideas in political policy making. These notions have been central in debates surrounding the future of public services. How services should be organised and to what extent users or clients should have a say in their running have been important in such debates. On the political right, the focus has been on the need for Citizens' Charters which specify 'rights' in terms of the type of service customers can expect to receive. This has seen a number of welfare providers and public (and private) utilities producing charters or statements of intent with regard to the services they aim to provide. Such political objectives have arisen due to the ideological stance of the New Right towards the importance of the individual in society (King, 1986). Individuals are seen as being disempowered by the State as they are not allowed to make choices about their own needs and wants (Barry, 1987). From this perspective, there is a need to ensure that citizens are free to pursue their own interests without State interference. This is done through increasing the role of the market in matters of choice, either by shifting State services from public to private ownership or by introducing business ethics and working practices into the publicly owned services. Both approaches claim to give more 'power to the people': customer satisfaction is guaranteed by the market as producers need to keep clients happy. Citizens' Charters are presented as methods of ensuring that individual needs and wants are catered for, giving people the right to complain if they feel that the services they receive are of poor quality.

The relationship between the citizen and public service providers has not been ignored by the political Centre and Left. The need to reduce the power of the State was initially tackled by policies of decentralising power to local communities (Blunkett and Green, 1983). A number of Labour authorities tried to shift control from the town hall to local communities by encouraging local people to be involved in decisions about how resources should be spent and distributed within areas. But in the face of legislative changes imposed by the Conservative governments in the 1980s and the massive restructuring of local finance, such an approach had little impact (Cochrane, 1989). In the 1990s, the Left remobilised its approach to empowering the citizen through campaigns such as those organised by Charter 88. One of the movement's central aims has been the need for the introduction of a Bill of Rights in which individuals have not only rights guaranteed *by* the State but also rights *against* the State, ensuring that individual freedoms and opportunities are maintained (Andrews, 1991). Such an approach has become important to Labour Party policy although it has refused to accept all of Charter 88's demands, suggesting that a Bill of Rights is taking the notion of a rights-based society too far.

These approaches of both Right and Left have major problems. As Taylor (1989) suggests, the New Right is more concerned with "consumer's than citizen's rights; with quality assurance, customer care and the rights of redress and exit" (p 19). Citizens' Charters in public services have little to do with the inclusion or exclusion of individuals from becoming full members of society. On the other hand, the development of a Bill of Rights as an approach to empowering the citizen ignores the fact that rights alone cannot challenge entrenched forms of social power. As Hall and Held (1989) suggest, rights fail to address the nature of social power in society and how certain groups are excluded by its exercise.

The research context of empowerment

Over the last few years, the concept of empowerment has also come to be of interest to the academic community. To begin with, there has been a growing demand for research methods which are sensitive to the ethical issue of exploitation of research subjects by researchers (Homan, 1991). Numerous disciplines have constructed practice guidelines which attempt to prevent such exploitation. For example, the British Sociological Association's statement of principles proposes that the researcher should "where possible attempt to anticipate, and to guard against, consequences for research participants which can be harmful" (1992, p 1). These guidelines therefore set a framework for ensuring that research should represent the views and experiences of participants in a manner that has the implicit potential for being empowering. As Homan (1991) has suggested, such an approach does have its problems. Codes of practice can have limited success in guaranteeing that professionals undertake their ethical responsibilities if the codes are ill-defined or lacking in professional sanctions (p 36).

A second area where the issue of empowerment has been raised is in feminist research. Since the late 1970s, the women's movement has raised the debate surrounding the purpose of research. Many have argued that research on and about women should be aimed at advancing women's issues and emancipation (Smart, 1977; Stanley and Wise, 1983; Ramazanoglu, 1992). Such arguments have suggested that research can have the objective of empowerment, ensuring that women's experiences and concerns are brought onto both the academic and political agendas, with the longer-term aim of improving the lives of women. This position has been criticised by writers such as Hammersley (1992) for failing to recognise the complexity of oppression and the subjective definition of need being used. Although, as Ramazanoglu states, Hammersley's criticisms seem to be based upon his assumptions about "what constitutes convincing knowledge [which] is rooted in the goals of science and rationality" (1992, p 207). Appeal to the rationality of science has dominated mainstream approaches to research methodologies and has historically marginalised concerns of the women's movement.

Third, the notion of empowerment has featured strongly in discussions concerning the role of research in contributing to the effectiveness of public services. Concern over the failure of services to meet users' needs has seen the development of research methods that give priority to the views of clients or users. Such an approach is not immune to ideological interests which may shape the way in which users are involved. At one level, empowerment is seen as being achieved through clients or users having a voice in the type and quality of service being given. This is then claimed as an effective method of evaluating public services. For example Cheetham et al (1992) identify the growing interest in this approach for evaluating social work. They suggest that this practice has evolved because of an awareness of the "negative effects of the early global attempts to demonstrate social work effectiveness" (p 31). Not all interests in this approach are stimulated by such concerns. Others have been prompted by issues such as 'value for money', efficiency and the need to satisfy external funders of their success[1]. Users' perspectives are elicited as a means of demonstrating whether services are achieving their aims at the most economic costs. Such a method is not empowering because it does not allow users control of the agenda or the questions being asked.

However, interest in the views of clients or users can be motivated by more genuine concerns about powerlessness. Croft and Beresford (1994) argue for users to be central in the organising of services not just to deal with issues of satisfaction, but also to examine issues of power (or the lack of it). They suggest that there have been two main approaches to user involvement: the 'consumerist' which, as we saw earlier, is associated with the New Right and which is manifest in Citizens' Charters, and the 'democratic' which is concerned with rights and self-advocacy (p 32). It is the democratic approach that supports the idea of service users speaking for themselves. As Croft and Beresford state: "Here the primary concern has been with empowerment, the redistribution of power and people gaining more say and control over their lives" (p 32).

Of course these debates over the ethics and purpose of research, and the importance of rights and self-advocacy in the development of services, are inter-related by their central concern with the powerlessness of those being researched. Academic debates about research methodology have introduced empowerment as a justifiable end to the research process (Reason, 1994).

In the following discussion, I will consider some of the dilemmas associated with putting a commitment to empowerment into practice in the context of an evaluation of Youth Action Projects (YAPs).

The national evaluation of Youth Action Projects

In 1993, youth services nationally were asked to tender, under Grants for Education and Training (GEST) funding for monies to develop locally based youth projects with the aim of developing ways of reducing young people's involvement in criminal and anti-social behaviour. Twenty-eight local authorities were successful and across the country projects were constructed with the central objective of targeting services on young people who were deemed 'at risk' of drifting into crime. Projects evolved around local needs and circumstances, giving each initiative its own uniqueness and individuality, although all schemes drew upon traditional youth work styles and methods. Funding was made available for three years with an overall budget of approximately £10m.

In 1994, Paul Wiles and I were contracted by the Department for Education and Employment (DfEE) to evaluate these projects. Our brief was clearly set in that we were asked to undertake two main objectives: a national audit of the projects, including identifying how the monies had been spent and what services had been developed, and an evaluation of the projects both in their own terms and those of the DfEE[2].

The research team proposed a methodology which was accepted by the DfEE that included a mix of quantitative and qualitative techniques. Commitment to a mixed approach reflected the consensus of opinion to emerge in the early 1990s which accepted that evaluation of youth work should be developed around qualitative methods (NYA, 1992).

Two main methods were highlighted for this evaluation. First, the research would involve two large surveys of all the projects with the aim of collecting and collating comparative data[3]. The second approach was the use of case studies. This entailed the identification of six projects that would provide in-depth insight into the day-to-day practices of the work being done. I was to visit the six selected sites for a week to investigate how each project had evolved, what methods it was using and how it was evaluating its work. This information would then be used in judging the overall success of the GEST programme as a method of crime prevention.

The idea that young people should be included in the evaluation of Youth Action was built into the original research proposal. Apart from the strong commitment of the research team to this ideal, it was felt that both the DfEE and youth workers would approve of young people having a say in the services they were receiving and about what they were getting out of the Youth Action programmes. Youth work has a long history in which questions of participation and empowerment have been important (Smith, 1988). As a method of working, youth workers claim one of their key aims is to empower young people. While the meanings and definitions of this have been much discussed, it is generally claimed by youth workers that empowerment "seeks to increase the control that young people have over their own lives and to increase the involvement they have individually and collectively in the decision making of agencies, institutions and systems in the provinces that affect them" (Kearney and Keenan, 1988). Such an ideal is clearly seen as central to the youth work curriculum. For example, in the Third Ministerial Conference on 'A Core Curriculum for the Youth Service' (NYA, 1992), it was decided that although a national curriculum was impractical because it restricted the expression of local needs, concepts such as empowerment, participation and equal opportunities should underpin the practice of the youth service.

This professional commitment of the youth service was a major influence in the acceptance of empowerment as a principle that should underpin our research methodology. The DfEE set up a steering group with the aim of supporting our work. This consisted of youth workers from the field, an inspector from the Office for Standards in Education (OFSTED), a representative from the National Youth Agency (NYA) and DfEE and Home Office civil servants. However, this group did not discuss either the principle or practice of empowerment. Youth workers appeared to have no concerns about empowerment because of their professional commitment, while civil servants expressed no interest. But this lack of discussion was also encouraged by me, as it was easier not to have to justify it to funders, or explain methods about which I was unsure. The research team had not devised empowering methods, and we were not clear about how we would implement and put such ideals into practice. Therefore, it was to our advantage not to engage in discussion about the meaning of empowerment. In sum, although a commitment to involving young people in the evaluation was built into the research proposal this did not mean that I had a clear idea about how this was to be put into practice. As the following discussion will show, this had major implications in terms of achieving such 'good intentions'.

It was the case studies which provided opportunities to involve young people in the research process and hence to implement our commitment to empowering methodologies[4]. As the projects were attempting either to challenge the behaviour of the young people or to improve their lives, it was felt that their experiences of being both involved in the projects and benefactors of services was an essential aspect of empowering them as users. But as mentioned by Croft and Beresford (1992), such a perspective is a limited notion of empowerment and does not necessarily give users greater understanding or control of their own lives. In the discussion that follows I explore how the methods used ran a fine line between empowerment and exploitation.

The case study evaluations and the involvement of young people

Due to the demands of the research timetable and because of the limited opportunity to spend time away from the university, the case studies had to be undertaken over a nine-week period. Much of the organisation and planning of the case study evaluations was undertaken on the telephone prior to the visit. It was necessary for youth workers in the different sites to be committed to the evaluation and to make the effort to structure a timetable for the week that would give access to individuals and settings that needed to be visited.

Case study one

The first visit was to an area-based YAP scheme. The project's main method involved youth workers in identifying a particular area or community in which crime was a problem, and targeting resources at groups of young people who were seen as being at risk of drifting into crime through contacts made on the street. The worker in charge arranged an evening session with a group of young people who had taken part in the project. The 'session' I attended consisted of arranging a trip to the local bowling alley. At this early stage, I believed this would provide a channel for young people to voice their own experiences about the local Youth Action Project, in turn giving them a voice in the national evaluation. I soon realised my failure to anticipate the potential hurdles associated with this approach. It became clear, at an early stage, that the youth worker had little idea about what I was trying to achieve. I had wanted to meet young people in a quiet and safe environment where they could talk openly about their experiences of being on the Youth Action Project. This did not happen. I met the young people while they were arranging the bowling alley trip in a minibus on a street corner. I had little control over how the session was to proceed and who was to be involved. Eventually I managed to get a small group of young people back to a local community centre to talk to them about their experience of the project. It was in this process that I then became aware of a second issue. As the session unfolded, it was clear that the young people had been primed by the youth worker. The following quote is taken from my field notes:

To start with it is worth saying something about the overall session. Jean had arranged it in advance and I felt that she had primed the young people about what I was coming for and what I was looking at. When we got talking they [the young people] spent some time trying to convince me they knew what the project was about. This had them arguing with each other, some claiming it was about keeping them off the streets and others saying it kept them out of trouble. I know they were primed because Jean kept trying to remind them in the mini-bus about what they should say.

The more I probed the more obvious this became. It was clear that young people were aware of the resource issues involved. They spent a lot of time convincing me that the money was being spent well and that it was stopping them getting into trouble. Clearly the youth worker had a stake in ensuring that I met young people who would report positive experiences of YAP. It was to the advantage of youth workers to demonstrate that the work they did was successful. Part of the reason for this arose because of the funding issue. Although all case study workers were reassured that funding and the evaluation were not linked, many may have felt insecure and attempted to protect themselves by producing young people who would support their claims of success.

The third issue that came out of this session concerned my ability (or inability) to manage the session and encourage young people to answer questions. As the session evolved, I had difficulty in keeping young people's interest and concentration. In many ways this was not surprising as they did not have any form of relationship with me. But this lack of interest may have arisen because the young people had little to gain from the session. I explained that I was there to find out what, if anything, they had achieved from taking part in the project. Young people saw that it was important to their youth worker to give positive responses to my questions about keeping out of trouble. But otherwise participation in the research meant little to them, as it was unlikely to improve their lives in the immediate future. The national evaluation and its purpose were unknown and young people had no stake in its success. Why should they make any real effort? The fact that young people took to 'messing about' – by talking among themselves and wandering around the room, for example – may therefore have been a method of rejecting the processes and structures imposed upon them by the evaluation, suggesting that instead of being empowering the research was in danger of exploiting young people's good nature and willingness to support their youth worker.

Case study two

The second case study differed from the first. Instead of working with groups identified on the streets, it took referrals from agencies such as schools and social workers. The young people were referred because these agencies deemed them to be having problems, such as academic difficulties at school, or to be a social problem in that they were regular truants or continually in trouble with the police and school authorities. The worker in charge organised a meeting with former members but this approach also had problems. First, only three young people turned up. Once again, young people had nothing to gain in talking to me about their involvement in Youth Action, so why should they be involved in my research? Another problem arose concerning their level of participation. Unlike young people in case study one, these ex-members had little to say. Getting them to talk about their experiences was far from easy. This was partly a result of their experience of Youth Action. Group work or group discussions had not been a feature of this project's method so young people did not know others in the group and/or feel at ease talking in a group setting. Feeling safe and being able to trust the person to whom they were talking was very important because the issues being discussed were personal and related to a time in their lives when they had either been in trouble or were having problems. Recounting this to a stranger with other strangers present was not something with which they seemed comfortable. This issue was clearly important and one that I needed to overcome if young people were going to have an active say in the effectiveness of YAP.

By the end of this case study I was becoming disillusioned with the attempts to involve young people in the national evaluation, feeling that maybe the methods had the opposite effect to this aim. Youth workers were clearly responding to my requests to meet young people but they appeared to be produced for my benefit. My impression was that young people's good nature and respect for their youth worker were being exploited to get a result for the research. It was at this point I attempted to change my approach.

Case study three

The third case study was of an area-based, detached project in which young people at risk of drifting into crime were identified by workers meeting them on the streets. Once young people were introduced to the project, they became involved in some form of informal education concerning matters that interested them or related to their needs. In this instance, I suggested to workers that I attend one of the project sessions, the aim being to approach the evaluation through observation and by meeting young people in a more natural youth work environment, though I insisted that they be consulted to see if they had any objections to my presence.

I was introduced to the group of young people at one of their planning meetings. They were discussing how their work on drugs information could be disseminated to other young people in the locality. This gave me an opportunity to join in and get participants to explain to me what they had been doing with the youth workers on the subject of drugs education. I was also able to ask how this related to their own lives and what they had learnt from the project. I introduced myself to the young people at the beginning of the session and briefly outlined the purpose of the national evaluation, although what they understood and saw as relevant to them was difficult to ascertain.

Whether such an approach was empowering is questionable due to the problematic issue of consent. Consent suggests choice, but did young people have real choice? Young participants were asked if they objected to taking part yet were they clear about what was being requested of them? How much choice did they really have? They had turned up that evening and been asked if they consented to me asking them questions, but would they have been so agreeable if they knew I wanted to probe into their private lives, if they had been asked the previous week and had time to reflect? Methods that focus on negotiated consent and use more personalised approaches may offer a better opportunity for involving young people. But it is important to recognise that power imbalances exist between young people and adults where they may not be able to say no. In these situations young people may be at risk of being exploited rather than empowered.

Case study four

As in case study two, case study four was a project that took young people who were referred from other agencies because they were seen as a social problem. Its method of working with young people differed in that, once referred onto the project, young people were introduced to a range of activities that aimed to be educational. It did not aim to intervene directly in the lives of young people or tackle the reasons why they were identified as a social problem. In contrast to case study three, I had to return to the format that had been set up prior to my visit. The workers invited a small group of past members to an after-school session. Having been through this process previously I decided to focus the meeting around the young people's experience of the project. To facilitate this, workers brought along photographs of activities in which members had participated. The aim was to encourage them to explain what the picture represented, how this experience reflected their time on the project and how it related to other aspects of their lives. Such a method was reasonably successful in getting young people to discuss their experiences of Youth Action, but similar problems to those of case study one and two still arose. Young people were unclear about what was being asked of them, while finding themselves among strangers in the group undermined their willingness to share in their personal experiences of Youth Action.

In this case study, a second opportunity arose to undertake some evaluative work with young people. It was agreed that I would go away on a residential weekend with the staff team and a group of young people. Residentials, as they are known, are regularly used by youth workers as a method of relationship building in which workers and young people can get to know each other by living closely together over a period of time. Participating in a residential thus gave me the potential to get to know a small group of young people in more depth. One of the difficulties with this approach was that the group of young people were a new cohort who had just joined the project and therefore their experiences and feelings about the project were going to be limited. But the experience helped me think about possible alternative approaches to involving young people in the national evaluation. It gave me an opportunity to overcome the problems of young people's lack of trust and uncertainty with the questioning. It also highlighted the importance of setting, once again showing relaxed environments are essential if young people's participation is to be encouraged. Residentials give ample opportunity to talk informally about more private issues and to express feelings and opinions about many issues. For example, the following abstract is taken from my field notes:

> **George was a lad that I got close to. He had been expelled over six times and excluded on a number of occasions. He said that he has no carpets in his house and that he has four other brothers. He talked to me about how he can and does lose his temper (has been to a 'special school' to try and learn methods of control) and about how he gets involved in criminal activities. He also talked about living on his estate and how this increased your chances of being a victim of crime. He said it wasn't uncommon to him to come home and get mugged of what little money he had.**

Such relationship building generated clear evidence that the Youth Action Project was focusing on young people who were at risk of drifting into crime. The problem was that because young people were new to the project it was not possible to have evaluative discussions.

By the time I had undertaken four case studies I realised that I had only been able to engage young people in a limited reflective evaluation. Empowerment remained elusive and ill-defined, and the methods had little to offer either young people or the national evaluation. Instead of continuing, I decided to discourage projects from assembling young people for my visits. I felt it was becoming an exploitative process in which they were produced as requested. This is not to say that I felt that they should not be included, but unless involvement was structured differently it was a pointless process that would be frustrating both to myself and the young people who were encouraged to take part in something about which they felt uncertain.

Conclusion

The central aim of this paper has been to show how good intentions, per se, are not enough when it comes to conducting research that claims to be empowering. It has also raised important issues concerning the construction of research approaches that are empowering within large-scale, government-funded, evaluative projects. The discussion has illustrated some of the difficulties that emerged when trying to empower young people who were defined, by the funding agency, as a social problem. This begs the question about the viability of participatory and empowering approaches within such research environments. As Barnes (1993) has argued, much social policy research which is funded by policy makers and designed by researchers can undermine attempts at empowerment. The requirements of funders to get answers to specific questions within tight time limits leads to a situation in which the funder effectively defines and sets the agenda. Empowerment, or the introduction of users' interests, into the construction of the research requires professionals to give up control and share power. Funders therefore have to learn to accept different disciplines and methods of evaluation (Barnes, 1993, p 39). This can challenge the control funders have because it threatens their professional roles and obligations. For example, those responsible for managing government funds may feel that responding to the concern of users and not ministers is alien to their professional culture.

As discussed earlier, challenges to the power base of professionalism may be taking place at the level of political discourse through arguments about how to create services that are more responsive to the needs of users. Yet such ideological shifts may only be at the level of policy making and not practice. Clearly, representatives for the DfEE were keen to support the notion of user participation and even empowerment included in the initial research bid, but their central concern was with providing outcomes for Ministers rather than empowering with users. Moreover, while concepts of empowerment and participation may well fit into the ideological and policy objective of 'consumerist perspectives', in terms of the organisational culture of the civil service and the traditional responses of Conservative Ministers to the youth crime problem, support for the notion of empowering young people remains open to question.

This being so, large-scale government-funded evaluative research may not be the best means by which to engage in empowering research. Political ideologies relative to user perspectives and involvement may be superficial at the level of practice within government departments. Such a perspective is worrying for researchers interested in developing more participatory and empowering approaches, but it is important to remember that the reason why this research struggled with the practice of empowerment related not just to a lack of commitment by funders but also to a number of other difficulties which were outside the influence of civil servants and politicians.

The growing support for consumerist or user perspectives provides opportunities to argue for more user-led research. In this context, the process of constructing the agenda and putting the research into practice has to address a number of other important issues from the very early stages of conception. The preceding discussion has identified a number of examples.

First, the notion of empowerment was seen as peripheral to the main objective of the research. It was also ill-defined, lacking any agreement by the relevant people involved about its value, as a research principle, to the focused area of study. What this experience tells us about doing research of this kind is that the acceptance of the principles of empowerment not only needs to be central to the methods devised but also clearly defined and discussed from the very beginning with all parties. If this does not happen then failure is highly likely.

Second, not only should the research agenda be openly debated between funders, researchers and gatekeepers from the beginning, but empowerment methods require that these initial discussions engage research subjects and allow them to decide what gains they desire from the research process. If empowerment means personal gain and positive improvement in participants' lives then we need to recognise what this means in practice and how it should influence the research design. A commitment to this approach therefore requires the development of methods that engage powerless people and give them opportunities to define the issues for themselves. These may comprise approaches which are not seen as conventional or do not fit neatly into the traditions advocated within the social sciences. For example, the case study work introduced here suggests that alternative methods such as the use of photography or life-experience discussions may be better approaches to engaging young people in talking about their feelings and needs than conventional semi-structured or group interviews.

Third and finally, researchers who claim to empower participants need to be aware of the different and complex set of power relations that may exist in the field. From the previous discussion it is clear that a number of different stakeholders influenced the research process and the objective of empowerment. The end result was that instead of young people being empowered they were being exploited because their involvement was aimed at meeting the needs of other stakeholders such as youth workers and researchers. This is not to blame other stakeholders, only to show how relationships of power can influence outcomes. What this suggests is that if the ideal of empowerment is to remain the central objective then there is a need to recognise that within the research process others may also feel disempowered and questions of empowerment may have either to tackle or at the very least recognise the complexity and divisions of power within the research process.

Notes

[1] For a discussion on the development of this approach in policy making see Pollitt, 1988.

[2] The final report on this research was published in September 1996: France, A. and Wiles, P. (1996) *The national evaluation of Youth Action Projects*, London: DfEE.

[3] The first of these would be undertaken at the beginning of the research and be repeated at the end of the second year of the programme. The surveys would serve to capture the process of change and development while also producing a national audit.

[4] The case study evaluations were constructed largely from qualitative data which was collected through semi-structured interviews, informal discussions and observations. The week-long visits comprised meeting and interviewing 'major actors' in each project, giving central focus to youth work staff, management and inter-agency partners. A series of questions relating to GEST objectives were devised, such as how the project was constructed, what its main objectives were and how it was measuring its success. The conclusions from these investigations were then to be fed into the national results as an important aspect of the evaluation.

References

Andrews, G. (ed) (1991) *Citizenship*, London: Lawrence and Wishart.

Barnes, M. (1993) 'Introducing new stakeholders: user and researcher interests in evaluative research. A discussion of methods used to evaluate the Birmingham Community Care Special Action Project', *Policy & Politics*, vol 21, no 1, pp 47-58.

Barry, N. (1987) 'Understanding the market', in M. Loney with R. Bocock, J. Clarke, A. Cochrane, P. Graham and M. Wilson (eds) *The state or the market: Politics and welfare in contemporary Britain*, London: Sage, pp 161-71.

Blunkett, D. and Green, P. (1983) *Building from the bottom: The Sheffield experience*, London: Fabian Society.

British Sociological Association (1992) *Codes of practice and ethical considerations of doing research*, London: BSA.

Cheetham, J., Fuller, R., McIvor, G. and Petch, A. (1992) *Evaluating social work effectiveness*, Buckingham: Open University Press.

Cochrane, A. (1989) 'Restructuring the state: the case of local government', in A. Cochrane and J. Anderon, *Politics in transition*, London: Sage, pp 95-140.

Croft, S. and Beresford, P. (1992) 'The politics of participation', *Critical Social Policy*, vol 2, no 2, pp 20-44.

Hall, S. and Held, D. (1989) 'Citizens and citizenship', in S. Hall and M. Jacques, *New times*, London: Lawrence and Wishart, pp 173-88.

Hammersley, M. (1992) 'On feminist methodology', *Sociology*, vol 26, no 2, pp 187-206.

Homan, R. (1991) *The ethics of social research*, London: Longman.

Kearney, D. and Keenan, E. (1988) 'Empowerment: does anyone know what it means?', *Lynx*, February, pp 3-5.

King, D. (1986) *The new right. Politics, markets and citizenship*, London: Macmillan.

NYA (National Youth Agency) (1992) *Towards a core curriculum for the youth service*, Conference Report, NYA.

Pollitt, C. (1988) 'Bringing consumers into performance measurement', *Policy & Politics*, vol 16, no 2, pp 77-87.

Ramazanoglu, C. (1992) 'On feminist methodology: male reason verses female empowerment', *Sociology*, vol 26, no 2, pp 207-12.

Reason, P. (1994) *Participation in human inquiry*, London: Sage.

Smart, C. (1977) *Women, crime and criminology*, London: Routledge and Kegan Paul.

Smith, M. (1988) *Developing youth work*, Milton Keynes: Open University Press.

Stanley, L. and Wise, S. (1983) *Breaking out: Feminist consciousness and feminist research*, London: Routledge and Kegan Paul.

Taylor, D. (1989) 'Citizenship and social power', *Critical Social Policy*, vol 26, Autumn, pp 19-31.

Having a say: involving young people in research on leaving care

Nina Biehal

The research context

Since the mid-1970s there has been growing concern about the vulnerability of young people leaving care arising from a number of related developments. First, the findings from a number of small-scale surveys and qualitative studies highlighted the loneliness, isolation, poverty, unemployment, homelessness and 'drift' experienced by many care leavers (Godek, 1976; Lupton, 1985; Stein and Carey, 1986; Randall, 1989). Second, from the mid-1970s young people in care began to come together to talk about their experiences. The self-organisation of young people in care, through the development of local 'in care' groups, the Who Cares? project, Black and in Care and the National Association of Young People in Care, also raised awareness of the connections between young people's experiences while in care and their lives after leaving (Stein and Ellis, 1983; Stein and Maynard, 1985; First Key, 1987). A third associated development was the reform of childcare law, beginning with the 'continuing care' recommendations of the 'Short Report' of 1984 (House of Commons Social Services Commission) and culminating in the 1989 Children Act, which gave local authorities new duties and wider powers to assist young people leaving care. All of the above developments led to the emergence of a range of local policy and practice initiatives designed to address the needs of care leavers which, by the mid-1980s, included the first specialist leaving care schemes.

It was in this context that my colleagues and I at Leeds University embarked upon a study of services for care leavers, funded by the Department of Health (see Biehal et al, 1995). The main purpose of our research was to evaluate four different leaving care schemes in three local authorities. Our aim was to improve our knowledge of the transitions made by young people leaving care in different areas of their lives – from (substitute) home to independent accommodation, from school to the labour market, from living with carers to living alone, with a partner or becoming a parent – and to evaluate the ways in which different types of leaving care schemes helped them to make these transitions. We decided upon a two-stage study, which began with a survey of patterns of leaving care in our three local authorities. Information was gathered on the transitions made by 183 young people and on the professional support available to them, by means of a postal questionnaire to social workers (Biehal et al, 1992). This was followed by an in-depth follow-up study of the process of leaving care and of the support offered to care leavers. Interviews were carried out with 74 care leavers, their social workers and, where applicable, specialist leaving care workers, on up to three occasions during an 18-24 month period after the young people left care. The second stage of the study enabled us to explore the social processes involved in leaving care and to evaluate the support offered by specialist leaving care schemes (see Biehal et al, 1995).

Although care leavers were not directly involved at the planning stage, the research design had been influenced by the perspectives of care leavers, based on two previous studies carried out by one of the researchers involved (Stein and Carey, 1986; Stein, 1990). Although involving care leavers in the research had not been one of the explicit aims of the study when it was first set up, once the study began it was rapidly agreed by all members of the research team that we should try to find ways of involving them. Although care leavers had not decided *what* should be studied – we were not besieged by care leavers clamouring for a study of leaving care schemes – we felt that it was essential to involve them in deciding *how* this study should proceed. If our aim was the evaluation of services, it was vital that the voices of the young people using those services should be heard. We hoped to involve them in setting the agenda for the study, in overseeing the study as it proceeded and in giving their views on their individual experiences of being looked after and of leaving care. Accordingly, we developed three strategies for involving young people in the research:

- involving care leavers in developing the questions the research would address through local discussion groups in the early stages of the study;
- asking care leavers to comment on and review the research as it proceeded, through the forum of regular project groups;
- interviewing individual young people shortly after they left care and on two further occasions over the following two years.

Why involve young people?

On a purely pragmatic level, we wanted to involve young people because this would lead to better research. Any evaluation of leaving care services which did not address the issues that service users considered important, and which did not fully explore the experiences of individual care leavers, would be of limited value. As researchers, we naturally wanted to produce good research, and this meant that users' views on the research design, and their experiences of leaving care, were necessarily central to the study. Clearly, in this respect, we were involving them in our own interests. Yet had we not attempted to produce the best possible research, our findings would be of little use to those developing services for care leavers and ultimately would have no chance of helping to improve services for these young people. If the research was to be useful to those leaving care in the future, it was particularly important for young people currently leaving care to be involved in setting its agenda and in defining the criteria for evaluating services.

A second, perhaps more fundamental, reason for involving young people in the research arose from our concern with the right of young people leaving care to be heard. Martin (1986) has indicated that the issue of user involvement in evaluation must be considered in the context of the welfare organisations in which it takes place, suggesting that these agencies typically place users in a weak position in relation to the organisation. The fact that users do not normally pay for services means that they have little power when it comes to determining what those services should be. As a group, they are likely to have little influence over the services offered locally and little choice. As individuals, their needs are likely to be assessed and defined for them on the basis of professional judgement, with the degree to which they are able to participate in defining their own needs contingent on local agency policy and practice and the personal approaches of individual professionals. Yet, as Barnes et al have pointed out, "the crucial question is, who defines the needs to which social services are asked to respond?" (Barnes et al, 1990).

Their weak position in relation to agencies providing services means that, in common with most other users of social services, care leavers are not in a position equivalent to consumers in the commercial world who have two options for expressing their dissatisfaction with a service or product – 'exit' or 'voice' (Hirschmann, 1970). If care leavers wish to 'exit' from services they consider unsatisfactory, they may be hampered by the twin constraints of economic disadvantage and the lack of alternative provision. 'Voice' is therefore the most straightforward way for users to express their preferences and their dissatisfaction. Yet, as Hirschmann has argued, 'voice' is often weak when 'exit' is not a realistic option. Although complaints procedures may be used to express individual grievances these, as Pfeffer points out, sometimes have the limitation that they close the door after the horse has bolted (Pfeffer and Coote, 1991). Individual voices giving their views on services may have little impact, but a research process which involves young people can assist a large number of users to bring their collective definitions of their needs to the attention of policy makers and practitioners.

Clearly, what lies at the heart of these debates is the question of power. Not only do these young people tend to lack power in relation to their use of social services, but also, more fundamentally, many of them have little power and opportunity to determine the course of their lives. Just as gender and poverty can combine to exclude women from full citizenship (Lister, 1990), poverty, age, and gender or 'race' may intersect to exclude some groups of young people. For care leavers, these factors are compounded by the fact that the majority are poorly equipped to enter the labour market due to low educational attainment and that many do not have access to the practical, emotional or financial support that families can provide (see Biehal et al, 1995). Unemployment, poverty, isolation and high rates of homelessness all combine to exclude many care leavers from full participation as citizens in the life of local communities, leaving them marginalised. The reasons for this are complex, deriving from a combination of the effects of separation from families and the experience of being looked after with the influence of social security policies and broader structural factors such as local and national youth labour and housing markets.

The fact that care leavers typically lack power both as citizens and as service users means that attention to their rights as citizens becomes particularly important for researchers. A central feature of our agenda, as researchers, was a concern with the rights of young people to be fully involved in decision making, both while they are looked after and when they leave care. As Croft and Beresford have suggested, the current concern with user involvement in social services may have implications for research, implying a more participatory approach to research as well as to practice (Croft and Beresford, 1988). Similarly, our attempt to involve young people in the research was directly associated with our concern with the rights of care leavers. However, while a participatory approach to practice may seek to empower service users, we could make no such grandiose claims for our tentative attempts to involve young people in research. Although we had no illusions that participating in the research would in itself be empowering to the young people, we were very clear that we did not want it to be a disempowering experience for them. We did not want this to be yet another occasion on which these young people felt they had little control over what was happening to them, or allow this to become an experience which might undermine their self-confidence and self-esteem.

Research that just takes from respondents can be exploitative. We wanted to offer something back, so that the research process might become more of an exchange (even though this was predominantly one-sided), both through involvement in the groups which helped to shape the research and within the interviews themselves. We hoped that the young people who became involved in the discussion groups and the project groups would gain through being listened to, having their views taken seriously, feeling they had a part to play in shaping a research study and developing transferable skills in participating in meetings. Nevertheless, although we recognised that our gains from their involvement were likely to be greater than theirs, future care leavers may ultimately benefit from the fact that these young people helped to shape the research process, helping to ensure that it was relevant to their concerns.

Setting the agenda

The purpose of both the early discussion groups and the ongoing project groups was to set the agenda for the research (although the project groups also had a wider rationale, to which I will return below). We wanted to know from the outset what issues and problems were important to young people currently leaving care and what questions they thought researchers should explore.

The discussion groups were set up at an early stage of the research and involved young people from the leaving care schemes. One-off meetings were held at the schemes' own project bases. On our behalf, scheme staff invited any scheme users who were interested to attend these discussions and also assisted us with providing transport where necessary. Practical assistance such as the provision of transport or childcare is essential if service users are to be involved in any forums such as these. As the young people were used to attending their schemes both for social events and in order to see their keyworkers, we thought they would feel most comfortable if we met on 'their' territory. Also, we hoped they would feel more confident and more in control of the discussion if they took part in it within a group that was familiar to them and where the researchers were clearly the outsiders.

We did not think it would be easy for the young people to think themselves into the position of researchers designing a study without any preparation. So we began by asking them what they thought were the main problems faced by care leavers and moved on from this to asking what kinds of professional help they had found more useful or less useful. Shifting from these discussions of concrete experience we then encouraged them to formulate a broader analysis of the needs of care leavers and how research might help to further their interests. We asked the young people, if *they* were commissioning research into services for care leavers, what would they like us to explore? If the ultimate aim of the research was to contribute to improving services, what information did they think we should gather to inform decisions about services for care leavers? In this way we tried to involve young people in developing the questions and hypotheses that the research would address. In the lively discussions which ensued the diversity of care leavers' needs and circumstances were reflected in the variety of agendas they thought we should address. The multiple and sometimes conflicting concerns they raised helped us to ensure that the research addressed the concerns of a wide range of care leavers.

The issues raised by these discussion groups informed the design of both our survey and our follow-up study and so had a real impact on the way the research proceeded. The discussion groups served primarily as a consultation process which we took very seriously, but we could not pretend that these groups gave young people direct control over the research agenda. We felt that control over the agenda of the research should more properly be shared between ourselves as researchers, care leavers and the local practitioners and managers of the schemes we were evaluating. Involving young people in the discussion groups was one means whereby we could hold ourselves accountable to care leavers and ensure that the research was relevant to their concerns, but we felt that we should also be accountable to the local agencies we were researching.

Collaborative research: involving young people in the project groups

In setting up the project groups in each of our local authorities, we hoped to involve both care leavers and those who directly provided services to them to ensure that the research was sensitive to local needs.

The project groups met twice yearly and included young people who had left care, leaving care scheme workers, social workers, residential and foster carers, managers, policy and research staff and children's rights officers. These groups served as a forum for developing approaches to the research, testing out research instruments, sharing problems and concerns and discussing initial findings. Our rationale was that the views of professionals committed to the interests of young people leaving care were as necessary to the research as the views of the young people themselves. We recognised that young people, scheme workers, social workers and managers all come from different power positions, but we also understood that while professionals are more powerful than the young people they work with, they themselves may lack power to change failings that they perceive in services. Practitioners may feel they have little control over the way services are organised or over the resources they can obtain for young people. It seemed important to us to work in collaboration with agency staff as well as young people, to ensure that the research was informed by the knowledge and experience of both groups and to ensure our accountability to both.

Involving young people in project groups where they were outnumbered by professionals was not without its problems, however. Groups composed of people from different power positions can inhibit the ability of those with the least power to participate effectively. If members of the group do not meet on equal terms, inexperienced group members may defer to those they perceive to have greater expertise or they may frame the issues to suit professionals (Richardson, 1983). Anxious to avoid the young people's inclusion in the groups amounting to little more than tokenism, we tried to develop strategies to make it easier for them to participate fully in these meetings.

The most simple and obvious strategy was to invite several young people along together, hoping that mutual support would give them greater confidence. However, it was difficult to ensure that a stable group of young people maintained their attendance and developed confidence, and sometimes only one young person would attend a meeting. The young people's fluctuating membership of the groups was partly due to the unsettled nature of their lives and partly due to their changing and developing interests. Not surprisingly, in view of the fact that the research extended over a four-year period, some moved away, some no longer identified themselves as care leavers and some simply lost interest.

Another very basic strategy was to keep the agendas and the conduct of the meetings informal and jargon-free. In one authority we also held some pre-meetings with young people just before the full meeting to give them an opportunity to discuss the issues on the agenda in advance, adding to them if they wished, and give them a chance to formulate their ideas in a smaller group which was composed of their peers. However, despite our attempts to facilitate their participation, all found it hard to intervene in meetings dominated by adult professionals. One young person explained that it was hard for him to 'jump in' to a discussion to make a point and said he would like to have direct questions addressed to him about his views.

Although the professionals at the meetings responded very positively to any contributions the young people made and demonstrated that they valued their opinions, we were concerned that the difficulties involved for them might leave the young people feeling undermined and less confident than before. However, feedback from some of the young people indicated that this was not the case and that they felt their views and experience were valued by others in the forum. Nevertheless, if we had possessed the resources to do so, we might have succeeded in engaging the young people more actively if we had held separate project groups for young people and professionals. On the other hand, there is clearly a great deal of value in helping young people to articulate their concerns to those who are more powerful. Both of these strategies require a major investment of time in order to prepare and support young people so that they can participate effectively in groups of this kind.

Interviewing young people

Seventy-four young people became directly involved in the research through agreeing to take part in interviews. We recognised that, as interviewers, we were potentially more powerful than the young people in two principal ways: within the interviewing relationship and in the way we used the information they gave us. In both cases, we were aware that it would be all too easy to exploit the young people. We were anxious to avoid this and we wanted to ensure that we protected their interests, both as individuals and as a group.

Feminist researchers have long been concerned with avoiding the potential exploitation of the subjects of research and have attempted to find ways of 'getting alongside' respondents as collaborators in a joint enterprise rather than maintaining the social distance between them (Stanley and Wise, 1983). Feminists have argued that detachment on the part of the interviewer in order to attain a degree of scientific objectivity – an approach that Oakley has dubbed 'hygienic research' – is neither desirable nor productive. As Oakley has argued, the maintenance of a hierarchical relationship between interviewer and interviewee should be replaced by "the recognition that personal involvement is more than a dangerous bias – it is the condition under which people come to know each other and to admit others to their lives" (Oakley, 1981, p 58).

In our shared commitment to the interests of care leavers we did not regard ourselves as detached from our interviewees, yet we recognised that our relationship with them was in many respects unequal. Differences in class, age and professional status inevitably put us in a more powerful position. We also had the power to interpret their accounts and formulate our own analyses of their experiences. Furthermore, each individual's account was to be interpreted not only in the context of the accounts of other young people, but also alongside the accounts given by professionals working with them. We wanted to be honest about exactly how their 'story' would be used and so explained to them at the outset that we wanted to look at their perspective on their experiences *alongside* the perspectives of the professionals working with them. We made it clear that in our 'pluralistic evaluation' no one's account would be privileged, we would not assume that either the young people or the professionals held the key to the 'truth' (Smith and Cantley, 1985). Rather, we accepted that accounts may not always fit together neatly and may sometimes be mutually contradictory. In our eventual analysis of the interviews we tried to represent competing narratives faithfully, while making it clear how we had come to our own interpretation of events and processes.

Recognising the imbalance of power between ourselves and the young people we interviewed, we felt it was most important to be honest with them in this way about exactly what their involvement would mean. Apart from assuring them that we would maintain total confidentiality and that we would disguise their names (and in some cases their circumstances) when writing up the research, we also made it clear that they would be unlikely to benefit directly from it. What we were asking of them was a degree of altruism, to share their time and their stories in the hope that the research might ultimately contribute to improving services for *future* care leavers.

As well as being clear about exactly what was involved, we tried to ensure that the young people were fully in control of their involvement in the research. To this end we initially approached them indirectly through their social workers or scheme workers, who gave them a letter explaining the project. If they agreed to take part we then wrote to them direct suggesting a time for an interview. This two-stage approach gave them two opportunities to refuse to take part before they first met us. We also took care to reassure the young people that we were completely independent of the social services or voluntary agency that they used and that their involvement in the research would in no way affect their access to services. At the end of interviews with young people we asked their permission to interview their social workers and scheme workers, and also asked if they would allow us to contact them again in few months for a further interview. In this way we tried to give them control over the extent of their involvement in the research at every stage. We also tried to give the young people a measure of control over the interview process itself by carrying out semi-structured interviews. The open-ended nature of the questions gave the young people greater scope to structure their narratives in their own way, with space to raise issues of particular concern to themselves.

Most of the young people we interviewed welcomed the opportunity to tell their story and it was not difficult for us to put them at their ease and establish a rapport. Yet the ease with which we could encourage young people to share their experiences with us raises questions about just how reciprocal the research relationship is. We were aware that the loneliness many of them experienced made them more than willing to talk to us. For some of the young people the interview provided a welcome opportunity to talk about themselves to a sympathetic listener, whereas our goal as researchers was to gather information. As Janet Finch suggests, the readiness with which more or less isolated people welcome the opportunity to talk about themselves in interviews does raise the question of whether the easiness and effectiveness of this style of interviewing with vulnerable or lonely people leads to exploitation (Finch, 1981). The fact that the interview may satisfy one set of needs for the researcher and another set of needs for the interviewee, to the mutual benefit of both if possible, should be openly recognised and great care must be taken not to exploit the vulnerability of lonely people. In a few instances, young people sought to use the interviews as a form of counselling, and it was necessary for us to be honest about the fact that we were not in a position to offer any commitment to a regular and continuing relationship of this kind.

However, we did feel that we had a clear responsibility towards the young people and did not want the interviews to constitute one-way exploitative relationships from which the researchers were the only ones to benefit. Where young people were clearly in need of help or advice, we explored with them at the end of the interview who might be the best person for them to talk to about the issues they had raised with us – social workers, leaving care scheme workers or specialist advice workers. We also tried to find other ways of giving something back to those we interviewed, even though we did not have the resources to pay them for their time. If, during the course of the interview, we discovered that they were unaware of their rights to a service or to a welfare benefit, we gave them the information they needed once the interview had ended. It seemed to us more important to repay them in any small ways that we could than to maintain detachment and methodological 'purity.' However, although we were aware of the vulnerability of many of the young people, we were anxious to avoid presenting them as victims when the research was written up. We tried to ensure that the resourcefulness and vitality of the young people we interviewed was apparent, and that we recorded their successes and developing strengths as well as their difficulties.

A logical extension of our strategy for involving young people in the interviews would have been to involve them in validating our findings prior to publication. At least two approaches are possible: first, to give individual care leavers the transcripts of the respective interviews we had held with them and second, to arrange for groups of young people who had been interviewed to comment on key findings and recommendations. Both of these approaches have methodological and resource implications. It would have been unreasonable to post transcripts to young people who had disclosed what was often distressing material to us, without being present to offer support as they read them, and time for discussion. In a study of 74 young people, which had already entailed over 400 interviews, this would have been prohibitively costly.

Organising the young people into groups to comment on key findings would also have been problematic, not least because it was extremely difficult to keep in touch with this highly mobile group, and it often took a long time to track down each young person![1] Also, it would have been unbalanced and unfair to do this without arranging parallel groups of social workers and leaving care scheme workers in each authority, requiring a massive investment of time and resources. More importantly, this raises the question of the status of respondent validation of this kind. As researchers, we felt our role was not simply to describe the views of various respondents but to offer an independent analysis of the varied perspectives of those we interviewed. If some of the young people had disagreed with our analysis, would it have been appropriate to have accepted their comments and changed our findings accordingly or should we have found some other way of incorporating these comments? It certainly would have been helpful for us to have had the opportunity to reflect on their comments before completing our final report and we could also have included an addendum to the report which directly expressed the young people's comments on our findings.

Both of these approaches would clearly provide opportunities for young people to be more fully involved in research, but the resource implications are massive and the methodological implications must be carefully considered. These are approaches that we would have liked to develop, but our failure to pursue either of these strategies had less to do with methodological concerns than with resource issues – the fact that we simply ran out of time as funding came to an end.

Involving young people in evaluating services

Attempts to involve young people in research raises wider issues about how the research is used and by whom. Apart from its potential usefulness for policy makers and practitioners, we need to be clear about which service users might find directly helpful. Here it is important to make a distinction between groups of users and the individuals who took part in the research. The latter would have been unlikely to benefit from any changes in service provision, given that in most cases their use of leaving care services is relatively short term (although on a personal level they may have enjoyed their involvement with the research). As suggested above, our intention was that the research might contribute to the development of services and thus benefit young people leaving care in the future.

However, the research might have been more directly useful to the young people who took part in it if there had been established user groups at each of the leaving care schemes. If this were the case, it would be easier to have a continuing dialogue with a group of service users, who could regularly comment on and help shape the progress of the research. An existing, self-organised group of this kind would be likely to feel more confident in developing their views – just as the young people found it is easier to contribute to our early discussion groups than to our project groups composed of young people and professionals. Two of the schemes had run young people's forums of this kind for a time, but both had come to an end before our study began. Both had been abandoned when they became dominated by what the schemes perceived to be a small group of more experienced young people, a situation which illustrates just how difficult it can be to put the rhetoric of user involvement successfully into practice.

It is also possible to involve young people in doing research which can more directly empower the young people carrying out the study and lead to a greater rapport between interviewer and interviewee, as well as providing a wealth of direct experience to inform the research design (Save the Children, 1995). However, like all approaches this is not unproblematic, raising a range of issues such as confidentiality, training and support.

If users are to participate effectively in the planning of services they need access to adequate information, and this is something that researchers can help to provide. If self-organised user groups are involved in research and help to shape its agenda and its progress, the end result should be research findings relevant to their concerns. These findings could be used to underpin a better informed dialogue between service users, policy makers and practitioners about the development of policy and practice. However, encouraging user involvement in research does have substantial cost implications if the users are to be properly prepared and supported to take part and also involved at a later stage in validating the research findings. Researchers and funding bodies who wish to encourage a participatory approach to research need to recognise and budget for the true costs of achieving effective involvement by users.

Acknowledgements
I would like to thank Jim Wade, Mike Stein, Nick Frost and Jasmine Clayden for their comments on earlier drafts of this paper.

Notes
[1] By the time of the final (third) interview, we were able to contact only 53 of the original sample.

References
Barnes, M., Prior, D. and Thomas, N. (1990) 'Social services', in N. Deakin and A. Wright (eds) *Consuming public services*, London: Routledge.

Biehal, N., Clayden, J., Stein, M. and Wade, J. (1992) *Prepared for living?*, London: National Children's Bureau.

Biehal, N., Clayden, J., Stein, M. and Wade, J. (1995) *Moving on. Young people and leaving care schemes*, London: HMSO.

Croft, S. and Beresford, P. (1988) 'Listening to the voice of the consumer: a new model for social services research', in M. Stein (ed) *Research into practice: Proceedings of the Fourth Annual JUC/BASW Conference*, Birmingham: British Association of Social Workers.

Finch, J. (1981) ' "It's great to have someone to talk to": the ethics and politics of interviewing women', in C. Bell and H. Roberts (eds) (1984) *Social researching. Politics, problems, practice*, London: Routledge and Kegan Paul, pp 70-88.

First Key (1987) *A study of black young people leaving care*, Leeds: First Key.

Godek, S. (1976) *Leaving care*, Ilford: Barnardos.

Hirschmann, A. (1970) *Exit, voice and loyalty. Response to decline in firms, organisations and states*, Cambridge: Harvard University Press.

House of Commons Social Services Commission (1984) *Children in care*, London: HMSO.

Lister, R. (1990) 'Women, economic dependency and citizenship', *Journal of Social Policy*, vol 19, pp 445-67.

Lupton, C. (1985) *Moving out*, Portsmouth: Portsmouth Polytechnic.

Martin, E. (1986) 'Consumer evaluation of human services', *Social Policy and Administration*, vol 20, no 3, pp 185-98.

Oakley, A. (1981) 'Interviewing women: a contradiction in terms', in H. Roberts (ed) *Doing feminist research*, London: Routledge and Kegan Paul.

Pfeffer, N. and Coote, A. (1991) *Is quality good for you?*, London: Institute for Public Policy Research.

Randall, G. (1989) *Homeless and hungry*, London: Centrepoint.

Richardson, A. (1983) *Participation*, London: Routledge and Kegan Paul.

Save the Children (1995) *You're on your own*, London: Save the Children.

Smith, G. and Cantley, G. (1985) 'Policy evaluation: the use of varied data in a study of a psychogeriatric service', in R. Walker, *Applied qualitative research*, Aldershot: Gower.

Stanley, L. and Wise, S. (1983) *Breaking out: Feminist consciousness and feminist research*, London: Routledge and Kegan Paul.

Stein, M. (1990) *Living out of care*, Ilford: Barnardos.

Stein, M. and Carey, K. (1986) *Leaving care*, Oxford: Blackwell.

Stein, M. and Ellis S. (1983) *Gizza say*, London: NAYPIC.

Stein, M. and Maynard, C. (1985) *I've never been so lonely*, London: NAYPIC.

Working with older people to evaluate the Fife User Panels Project

Marian Barnes

Introduction

The Fife User Panels Project is described by Joyce Cormie elsewhere in this collection (pp 27-38). Its aims were to enable frail older people to discuss with each other their experiences of growing older and of using health and social care services, and to use the outcomes of such discussions to influence the provision of services to become more sensitive to older people's needs. At the time the project was developed there were few examples of frail older people being involved in community care planning. Thornton and Tozer (1995) reviewed initiatives across the UK which sought to give a voice to older people. They described the Fife project as having 'broken new ground' in enabling frail older people to meet together over time to talk about community care. In view of the significance of the Fife project as a potential model for other initiatives to involve frail older people it was agreed from the start that the project should be evaluated and separate funding was obtained for this purpose. I acted as consultant to the project, drawing on experience of working in a similar way with carers (Barnes and Wistow, 1993) and was also responsible for coordinating the evaluation. In this paper I consider one aspect of that evaluation: working with older people not involved in the panels who volunteered to interview panel members about their involvement. The results of the complete evaluation are reported elsewhere (Barnes and Bennet-Emslie, 1997).

The evaluation

The evaluation was designed to answer three questions:

1. First, is it possible to identify frail older people who are, or could be, users of health and social care services, and to involve them in regular panel meetings designed to encourage them to articulate their views about such services? This basic "Is it possible?" question was prompted by evidence of scepticism about the feasibility of the initiative when it was first proposed. It was questioned whether frail older people would want to engage in regular meetings which might be quite physically demanding. Questions were also asked about the likely 'representativeness' of panel members; and whether all group members would contribute equally to discussions, that is, would the voices of the most frail really be heard?

The importance of the issue of 'representativeness' prompted the project workers and me to write a paper on this topic early in the project (Barnes et al, 1993). In this paper we distinguished between three different meanings of the term 'representative':

- the notion of a representative sample referring to the extent to which a sample deliberately selected by a researcher can be considered to represent a known population;
- the notion of an individual or individuals, who can be elected to represent and be accountable to a particular constituency without necessarily sharing any of the characteristics of other members of that constituency;
- the sense in which the experience of particular individuals can be considered to be typical of those of many others in a similar situation and thus may 'represent' a wider experience by example.

It is this third meaning which we considered the most appropriate to apply in the case of the User Panels Project.

Monitoring data was kept by the project team to enable an analysis of the characteristics of the older people who were nominated as potential panel members and of those who subsequently agreed to become participants. Information about attendance and reasons for non-attendance or for leaving the panels was also recorded. Detailed notes of meeting discussions and the methods used to encourage discussion were kept to enable an analysis of group dynamics and of the way issues were raised.

2. The second question posed by the evaluation was: "Do older people experience benefits from being involved in such panels?" This was prompted by earlier experience of user involvement initiatives which suggested that, since service development outcomes are both uncertain

and require a considerable time period before they are likely to be demonstrated, some intrinsic benefit from participation is important in order to ensure continued motivation to participate (Barnes and Wistow, 1993; Barnes, 1995b). The interviews discussed here aimed to explore panel members' views about the experience of being involved. In addition to these interviews, panel members were also interviewed by project staff using a structured schedule before becoming members of the panels and at two points during the three years of the project, to assess whether there had been any change in their sense of control over important aspects of their lives.

3. Although service development outcomes are likely to be limited in the short term, nevertheless a major objective and justification for the project was that it would lead to changes in services. Hence the question: "Do the panels exert any influence over service plans and provision?" was the third one to be posed in the evaluation. In order to explore this question an independent researcher was appointed to 'track' three key issues which emerged early on as being problematic for panel members. These three issues were: access to information about services and methods of making complaints about services; domiciliary care services; and hospital discharge. The latter has been discussed in more detail elsewhere (Barnes and Cormie, 1995).

The tracking of responses to these issues involved interviews with key informants among health purchasers and providers and within the social work department; analysis of communications between panel members and the statutory agencies; and analysis of internal documentation relevant to the three issues produced prior to the panels being established and after they had started raising the issues.

Older people interviewing older people

The project philosophy was that older people have been active participants, either in work, families, voluntary work, politics or other social activities, and they continue to be capable of active participation in determining how services should be provided in order to meet the needs associated with their frailty.

It was considered important to extend that philosophy to the evaluation – to see older people not as 'experimental subjects', but as participants in designing and conducting the evaluation. Both the theory and practice of participative research have seen substantial development during the last 10-15 years (see for example Beresford, 1992; Barnes,

1993, 1995a; Reason, 1994). Not only have users of services sought to become involved in decision making about those services, they have sought to become involved in designing and undertaking their own research. This has been seen to be important in its own right as a means of reclaiming a right to self-definition and determining the nature of the 'problem' to be studied (Oliver, 1987), and as a means for increasing their influence over service content and design (Beeforth et al, 1990).

While the evaluation of this project cannot be considered as an example of research controlled by users, it did involve older people in the process of designing the study as well as participating in carrying it out. In the remainder of this paper I will describe how I and the project staff went about this and discuss the queries I have about the way we did this and what alternative methods we could have used.

In addition to the objective of involving older people as participants in the process of evaluation, three factors affected our decision about the particular methods we employed:

- We decided on individual interviews rather than group discussions with panel members in order to explore their experiences. This was intended to draw out differences in members' responses to the experiences as well as identifying common themes. It was in part a response to attitudes we encountered within local health and social care agencies towards the panels: it was intended to allow the individual voices of panel members to be heard through a different means to that offered by the panel meetings themselves. Also, by the time the interviews were being planned most of the panels had been meeting for more than a year and reports from project workers indicated that, while groups were working well together, there were indications of different expectations and responses to the operation of the panels which we thought it would be important to explore.
- By definition, the panel members are very frail. They cannot travel without assistance and some require considerable assistance to get ready to attend panel meetings. If interviews were to be conducted in their own homes we needed to involve older people who were physically more capable of travelling under their own steam than the members themselves. In other words, we wanted to involve older people as interviewers, but they would not be people who would meet the criteria for involvement in the panels.
- I had realised through my involvement with the project that language was an important issue. Some of the words I used did not mean quite the same thing in Fife, and some of the words local people

used were not familiar to me. For example, the term 'being a bother' to someone was used frequently by panel members. While I understood what this meant, it was not a term I naturally used. Because terms such as this are value laden I thought it would be better to ask older people living in Fife to conduct the interviews because they would share a language with those they were interviewing. Subsequently I discovered that many of the panel members don't come from Fife, and neither did some of those recruited to do the interviews! Nevertheless, the decision to use older people living locally was intended to maximise the possibility of empathy between interviewer and interviewee in terms of both language and experience.

The interviewers

Six volunteers were involved in both the design and conduct of the interviews. One was a member of the local advisory group established to oversee the User Panels Project, and another worked as a volunteer for Age Concern in the area. The other four were personal contacts of project workers. All were over retirement age, with ages ranging from the late 60s to the 80s. Five of the six were women.

The two volunteers who worked with Age Concern probably had the best idea of what would be involved before they started. The others were motivated, I suspect, partly by the fact that they were asked by people they liked and respected, and partly by curiosity. As we discovered, this reflects some of the reasons why older people became involved in the panels themselves (Barnes and Bennet-Emslie, 1997).

The process

I met with volunteers on three occasions during the course of a week in order to prepare the interview schedule and to introduce them to the practicalities of undertaking research interviews. Each session took place in a meeting room of a centrally located community centre. Where necessary, volunteers were given lifts to the sessions and those who travelled under their own steam had their expenses paid. All three sessions took place during the morning and ended with lunch.

The sessions involved the following:

Session 1

The project worker described the User Panels Project for the benefit of those who had no previous knowledge of it. She then conducted a role-play in order to give the volunteers a flavour of the processes involved in the panel meetings and the types of issues discussed:

- What do you feel about getting older?
- What are the good things about it?
- Is it more difficult to get things done?
- Do people take as much notice of you?
- Do you find it easy/difficult to complain when you're not satisfied?
- Do you meet up with people your own age?
- Do you feel more dependent on others?
- With what sort of things do people seek your help/advice?
- What do you make of health services etc?

I then asked the volunteers to reflect on the experience of discussing those sorts of issues in a group: was it an unusual sort of thing to have done? How did it make them feel? What did they enjoy about it? Was there anything that they felt uncomfortable about? What might they want to gain from being involved in such a process? I took notes both of the discussion and of volunteers' response to this.

Next, I introduced the evaluation, describing the reason for doing it, the three questions it was addressing, who was involved in the evaluation and how I saw the role of the volunteer interviewers within it. At the end of the session I asked volunteers to think about whether they wanted to continue now they knew more about what was involved. I finished by suggesting that I should take away my records of the discussions and come up with an initial draft of an interview schedule for them to look at and comment on at our next meeting. This was agreed.

Session 2

On the second day I recapped on the previous session and confirmed that they all wanted to continue. We looked at the draft interview schedule which I had prepared the previous afternoon and considered:

- Were the questions the right ones?
- Would it be useful to add any other questions?
- Was the wording easily understandable?
- Would volunteers feel comfortable asking them?
- Would they feel comfortable answering them?

A few amendments were suggested and I took note of these to incorporate the changes in time for the next session.

The volunteers then worked in pairs to role-play administering the schedules which included practice of note taking during the course of the interview. Each took it in turns to be interviewer and interviewee while I observed and made suggestions where necessary.

We discussed any problems volunteers had experienced and considered how they might be resolved, for example, how to encourage fuller responses if people gave only one word answers. I undertook to make further revisions to the schedule for the final session as well as to come up with a draft letter to be sent out in advance to interviewees.

Session 3

The final session was mainly concerned with the practical and procedural requirements of conducting the interviews. Project staff were to be responsible for the administration arrangements and this needed to be coordinated between the office and the interviewers. We looked at the introductory letter to be sent out notifying panel members that the interviews were taking place and volunteers suggested some amendments to this. We also discussed further issues relating to the conduct of interviews, including:

- factors which might affect the way in which interviews would need to be conducted, for example, hearing or sight problems;
- factors which would affect when it would be a good time to arrange the interview, for example, what time the district nurse called, or how long it took people to get up in the mornings;
- arranging to visit someone in their own home and creating a situation in which the interviewee feels relaxed and comfortable and the possibility of interruptions is minimised;
- focusing on people's views without making them feel as if you're interrogating them;
- dealing with their questions to you;
- leaving.

We also discussed the importance of more technical matters:

- ensuring that the code number was recorded on the interview schedule and the tape so that they could be linked when the analysis was conducted;
- recording responses in a way which made it clear when these were verbatim and when the interviewers' summary;

• checking through notes after the interview to ensure they were legible.

Finally, we agreed a date when we would get together after the completion of the interviews to discuss volunteers' experiences of conducting the interviews and to consider initial findings from them.

Issues from the introductory sessions

Involving volunteers did make a difference to the content of the interview schedule. Before the introductory sessions, I had prepared possible questions based on previous work I had done with carers' panels (Barnes and Wistow, 1993) and my knowledge of the Fife User Panels. Both the content and wording of questions changed as a result of the discussions with volunteers. For example, one issue which emerged in discussions to which I had made no reference concerned the assumption that older people would want to meet in groups with other older people. The final schedule included questions designed to explore whether panel members might see any benefit in participating in groups involving people of different ages. Another issue, which emerged during a discussion of volunteers' responses to their experience of talking about how they felt about growing older, was the potential significance of demonstrating a natural interest in other people's lives. It was considered this might counteract concerns that discussing personal experiences in a group might be intrusive and the interview schedule was amended to explore what panel members themselves thought about this.

The discussion also identified criteria which could be specified when considering the potential benefits or disbenefits of involvement. These were included as 'tick box' sections which would allow direct comparison between responses of interviewees.

Only one of the volunteers knew anything about the panels before these sessions and all were very interested in the idea. Some asked if they themselves could go along to panel meetings. This provided a direct demonstration of potential value which older people see in such opportunities. In the course of the role-play panel discussion some participants found out information about local resources of potential value to themselves. Information sharing was an important intrinsic benefit identified by carers who participated in the Birmingham Carers' panels (Barnes and Wistow, 1993) and this experience confirmed that this is likely to be a general benefit of this model of group working. To the extent that information about services can enable people to be more assertive in seeking access to sources of assistance, this can be seen as an empowering outcome in its own right.

However, in one important respect I did not think that our objectives were met. One purpose in working with older people as volunteer interviewers was the potential for them to develop new skills. None of the volunteers had done any research interviewing before, although one who had been a speech therapist had been used to visiting people at home to assess them, and another was a voluntary visitor for Age Concern Scotland and thus was used to talking with people in their own homes. The role-play demonstrated a common problem experienced by people administering structured interviews for the first time: the tendency to pose questions in an unnatural voice in a way which inhibits the free flow of conversation. The natural communication abilities of the volunteers may have been *constrained* by the use of a structured schedule, even though they had been involved in its design. The volunteers demonstrated little apprehension about going out to visit people, but were more concerned to do things in the way that was being asked of them. One said, "You're asking an awful lot of us". In this respect it is uncertain that they gained any new skills which were likely to be helpful to them in other parts of their lives. I return to this issue below.

Feedback after the interviews had been conducted

Before I met with the interviewers after the interviews had been completed I had undertaken an initial analysis of results, based on notes taken by interviewers, but not transcripts. Thus the three purposes of the feedback meeting were:

1. to obtain interviewers' perspectives on the content of interviews;
2. to provide an initial response to the draft report;
3. to consider experiences of conducting interviews.

Here I focus on their experience of conducting the interviews.

One person had experienced difficulty getting more than yes or no answers from interviewees. She was worried about this in terms of not having collected sufficient information for the evaluation, and somewhat disappointed that she had not found the experience a more engaging one. It was suggested that the people she interviewed might have been less likely to open up than some of the other panel members, but the interviewer herself thought she would have got a lot more information if she had just sat and had a chat about the panels, rather than going through the schedule. Other interviewers made a related point. They felt that they would have got more out of the interview if they had been able to go back twice – the first visit to establish a relationship with the person they were interviewing and to find out more information about the panels, the second to explore in more detail what people thought about them.

All said they were well received. They were offered hospitality and in some instances tea and biscuits were set out in advance ready to be served to them. Interviewees recognised the need for a hard surface to write on and ensured that it was possible for the interviewer to have a chair next to a table for this purpose. Interviewers received a number of invitations to return to visit on another occasion and one interviewer was obviously touched to have received a letter from the woman she interviewed expressing pleasure at her visit. None felt awkward or embarrassed asking the questions and none found it a problem to write answers down as they were conducting the interview.

The interviewers did not consider that being local people of similar ages made a difference to their ability to communicate effectively with interviewees. They felt that anyone going in prepared to chat to 'make a bridge' and to treat the interviewees sympathetically would have established the sort of relationship necessary to conduct the interviews. Overall they enjoyed doing the interviews, although some had experienced difficulties because of the bad weather and suggested that it might have been rather more enjoyable in summer. They felt they had learnt from the opportunity to find out more about the panels and what members thought was important about them.

Conclusions

The decision to use structured interviewed schedules was made because the interviews were to be conducted by six different people, none of whom had previous experience undertaking research interviews. The aim was to ensure consistency and comparability in order to generate results which would be considered valid by those assessing whether the User Panels Project had been a useful and effective way of engaging with older people to explore their views about services.

If I had been conducting the interviews myself I would not have used such a structured approach. I would have used a series of headings as prompts to ensure that I covered all the topic areas, but I would have aimed to develop the interview in a naturally flowing manner, rather than following a predefined series of questions. I'm increasingly convinced that structured interview schedules do not enable responses as rich as those which can be gained from less formal means – in particular if the interviewees are people who may be unused to being in such a position or uncomfortable with it. I was very aware recently when interviewing someone who had been a user of mental health services that, although I was trying to adopt an informal style, he still associated being asked questions with being 'assessed' or 'diagnosed'.

Perhaps I was insufficiently confident that the volunteers would be able to adopt a similar unstructured approach to interviewing while still covering all the topics we had agreed were important. Perhaps if it had been possible to have a longer period of preparation together I might have suggested this approach. But my conclusion is that I was probably paying more attention to meeting the expectations of those we hoped to influence through the evaluation than I was of the skills which the interviewers brought with them to this exercise and which could have been more effectively employed.

Working with older people made a difference to the questions asked and provided a direct demonstration of some of the advantages of the panel model. But the use of a structured schedule may have inhibited responses and, rather than helping them to develop new skills, did not enable interviewers to make use of their existing communication skills to explore the responses of panel members in as much depth as may have been possible using a less structured approach.

The aim of maximising sympathetic relationships between interviewers and interviewees appeared to have been successful. However, the assumption that rapport would be assisted by 'matching' interviewees with interviewers of a similar generation living in the same area was questioned by the interviewers. Some local knowledge provided an opportunity for conversation to 'build a bridge', but this was not considered essential. However, after listening to the recordings of interviews, I think I would have found at least one interview difficult to conduct because of my difficulty in understanding the accent and language.

While this exercise clearly demonstrated that older people can participate effectively in the conduct of research, both caution and time constraints may have limited the extent to which that participation shaped the conduct of this element of the evaluation. Nevertheless, the volunteers enjoyed their involvement and said they would be prepared to do it again. It also provided an opportunity for information about the User Panels Project to be spread more widely (among volunteers and their contacts) and indicated that interest in the possibilities offered by the panels could extend beyond current panel members.

References

Barnes, M. (1993) 'Introducing new stakeholders: user and researcher interests in evaluative research. A discussion of methods used to evaluate the Birmingham Community Care Special Action Project', *Policy & Politics*, vol 21, no 1, pp 47-58.

Barnes, M. (1995a) 'Evaluating user and carer involvement in community care', in J. Waterson and M. Bernard (eds) *Working together. User and carer involvement in community care*, University of Keele: Evaluation Research Unit.

Barnes, M. (1995b) 'Partnerships in research: working with groups', in G. Wilson (ed) *Community care: Asking the users*, London: Chapman and Hall, pp 228-41.

Barnes, M. and Bennet-Emslie, G. (1997) *'If they would listen...'*, *An evaluation of the Fife User Panels*, Edinburgh: Age Concern Scotland.

Barnes, M. and Cormie, J. (1995) 'On the panel', *Health Service Journal*, 2 March, pp 30-1.

Barnes, M., Cormie, J. and Crichton, M. (1993) *Seeking representative views from frail older people*, Edinburgh: Age Concern Scotland.

Barnes, M. and Wistow G. (1993) *Gaining influence, gaining support: Working with carers in research and practice*, Leeds: Nuffield Institute for Health, University of Leeds.

Beeforth, M., Conlan, E., Field, V., Hoser, B. and Sayce, L. (eds) (1990) *Whose service is it anyway? Users' views on co-ordinating community care*, London: Research and Development for Psychiatry.

Beresford, P. (1992) 'Researching citizen involvement: a collaborative or colonising exercise?', in M. Barnes and G. Wistow (eds) *Researching user involvement*, Leeds: Nuffield Institute for Health, University of Leeds, pp 16-32.

Oliver, M. (1987) 'Re-defining disability: some implications for research', *Research, Policy and Planning*, vol 5, no 1, pp 9-13.

Reason, P. (ed) (1994) *Participation in human enquiry*, London: Sage.

Thornton, P. and Tozer, R. (1995) *Having a say in change: Older people and community care*, York: Joseph Rowntree Foundation.

Conclusion: empowerment: the path to partnership?

Lorna Warren

Introduction

Empowerment has been declared the driving force within contemporary UK health and social services (DoH, 1991). The problem is that the concept is an 'elusive' (Hollingberry, 1994) and a 'contested' one (Means and Lart, 1994b). The complexity is evidenced by varying terminology. Recent policy change emphasised the need to stimulate 'choice' for service users (DoH, 1989). But the idea that users could exercise a 'voice' about the services they receive appeared much earlier (Mayer and Timms, 1970). In the ensuing period, commentators have employed other terms such as 'involvement', 'participation' and 'partnership'. The terms have been criticised variously as being "too vague", for "suggesting an equality which is rarely possible", or for drawing from social and political frameworks such as the consumerism debate with which professionals (and also users) do not necessarily agree (Stevenson and Parsloe, 1993).

This chapter – presented initially as one of the papers in the Sheffield seminar series – acknowledges and explores some of the reasons for the confusion, elusiveness and contestation. It was stimulated by two main issues. From a personal perspective, I had been aware for a long time of a tension between my thoughts on empowerment and my experiences of conducting research in this area, the development of the former often out-pacing the practice of the latter.

In this chapter I demonstrate the futility of trying to produce a single notion of empowerment which is recognised, instead, as an "evolving *process*" (Stevenson and Parsloe, 1993). I illustrate how and why different actors may be involved in various ways and to various degrees in empowering processes. I set empowerment issues for users and for carers alongside those for professionals and researchers, highlighting the necessity of addressing a range of concerns in order to build alliances and partnerships.

Perhaps a more immediate spur for writing the paper was the observation made by a colleague that the Participation and Empowerment research group within the Department of which we were members had at no point actually attempted to sit down and discuss what the terms 'participation' and 'empowerment' meant to us. In setting up this seminar series, the group had given speakers the freedom to approach their presentation from the direction of their choice. Contributors not only used and added to the terms collectively embracing user empowerment – referring in addition, for example, to consultation and representation – but encompassed a wide range of activities and perspectives in the process.

My aim, then, was to review a number of these presentations and the ensuing discussions with participants at the seminar series and the Working in Partnership workshop (see Introduction), with additional reflections on my own experience as well as the wider literature. I chose to focus on the accounts and visions of various groups, including professionals and researchers as well as users, carers and members of the wider community, which were currently or potentially directly involved in empowering processes, rather than on theoretical considerations of models of empowerment which have been well documented elsewhere[1].

My review concentrates on the presentations which form the contributions to this book and which were derived from the first in the three rounds of the seminar series. The review is perforce selective. I have not, for example, reflected the perspectives of people with learning difficulties among whom general progress towards participation is relatively widely developed (Whittaker, 1990; Simons, 1994). Neither do I talk specifically about people with a mental illness, whose involvement in self-advocacy groups is increasing steadily (Campbell, 1993), or young people, whose right to be heard has been traditionally weak since they typically lack power both as citizens and as service users (Biehal, 1993). Brian Davey's contribution on deprived communities and Adrienne Wright's on user forums within an NHS trust are both developed from their respective experiences of working with mental health user groups, although both have wider relevance. Nina Biehal's and Alan France's discussions of the research process focus on particular groups of young people, but cannot be considered to represent the views of young people themselves. I have drawn on the literature to include discussions of the perspectives of carers and professionals since, although carers do not feature as the specific subject of any of the chapters and professionals as a central focus of only one (see Wright), members from both groups did form a significant presence in the audience.

Participants in empowerment: users, carers and community groups

Disabled people

Disabled people have one of the strongest profiles in terms of the proactive pursuit of civil rights. Nevertheless, Ken Davis describes the 'gulf' which still remains between the movement's definition of disability as social barriers preventing participation in mainstream society on equal terms, and community care's authoritarian paternalistic perception of disability as an individual problem requiring paid officials to define, classify, register and control. Indeed, one participant at the workshop noted the "disruptive", "soul-destroying, totally negative experience" of the review process for benefits:

> **Because the person that comes to do it doesn't know anything about that person very often. The country is paying a doctor, who is a stranger to the family and a stranger to the disabled person, to come and carry out the investigation and the person who is being reviewed and their family sometimes feel that they've got to paint the greatest possible black picture in order that their allowance can be continued.**

This is not to deny the existence of opportunities for disabled people to gain influence. In initiatives such as the Living Options scheme in east Devon (Swain, 1993)[2] or Margin to Mainstream in Sheffield and elsewhere (Goss and Miller, 1995)[3], informal confederations representing disabled people have been established which have aided collaboration with statutory and voluntary agencies. The Independent Living Fund was closed in 1993[4] but, in 1997, the Direct Payments Act was passed enabling councils to give individual disabled people the cash to buy their own services, albeit with restrictions and as a discretionary power rather than a duty.

Yet numerous barriers to the involvement of disabled people in community care planning at the wider policy level still remain, including: lack of consultation with disabled people before preparing draft plans; inaccessibility of plans to people with learning difficulties; lack of payment of users for their time; the exclusion, alienation, or marginalisation of user representatives within meetings; the questioning of representativeness far beyond that of other interest groups; and the insufficient recognition of the unfriendliness of planning structures (Bewley and Glendinning, 1992). At an even more basic level, offering disabled people the opportunity to participate in consultation meetings is a thwarted exercise while services are only available to people in their own home and do not include transport or escorts to help them to go out (Morris, 1994a). This situation plays a role in the development of what the convenor of the workshop, Jonathan Swift, referred to as the 'professionalisation' of users (and carers): that is, the repeated use of the same individuals to talk about their experiences or to give their views on services. The phenomenon implies token efforts at reaching out to users on the part of professionals, as well as risking the exhaustion of individuals who do make efforts to be heard.

On the other hand, not all disabled people necessarily seek collaboration with service providers. Disabled people's self-organisation has, in many instances, taken an approach to empowerment that goes beyond consumerist philosophy to focus on the citizenship of disabled people (Barnes et al, 1996; Barnes, 1997). But governments have clearly been reluctant to cede influence beyond the planning process: key elements of the 1986 Disabled Persons (Services, Consultation and Representation) Act covering local authority services for disabled people have never been implemented, and attempts to give disabled people legal protection against discrimination in the alternative form of a comprehensive Civil Rights (Disabled Person's) Bill have been repeatedly blocked. The recent government 1996 Disability Discrimination Act, which makes it unlawful to discriminate in employment and the provision of goods and services, has been criticised for being a 'piecemeal measure', with definitions of disability that are a 'shambles' and which essentially will be a lawyers' charter[5] (Barnes and Oliver, 1995). Moreover, as Ken Davis notes, new tensions are arising in 1998 because of the slow progress on comprehensive civil rights legislation, and also as a result of the lack of clarity of new Labour's intentions regarding welfare reform.

Many believers in the social model of disability support the notion of a self-help disability movement which can bring together *all* oppressed and marginalised groups in challenging the existing political system (Oliver, 1990; Morris, 1991). Their argument is that separate consideration of different care groups reinforces the medical model, masking the disabling character of society and much social policy. But, while users may be united by shared experience of forced dependency and a common goal of empowerment, it cannot be assumed that individuals agree about the identity to adopt in order to fight for that goal or the path of the battle: for example, some people reject the term 'disabled' as a stigmatising label, others object to the degree of emphasis placed on physical access by the disability movement.

Older people

Despite the publication of the Age Concern *Manifesto* (Age Concern, 1974) and the actions of other voluntary organisations in speaking on behalf of older people, older people have not achieved the same kind of strength or prominence as disabled people in organising and speaking out for themselves.

At the wider political level, a single-minded organisation of ten million people is very unlikely given wide-ranging differences in class, age, gender, ethnic status, family circumstances, and political involvement in the past. People may be unwilling to be labelled 'old', especially if they have joined this category as a result of redundancy and enforced retirement. They may feel that because they cannot withdraw their labour, they have no effective sanctions (Hobman, 1994).

In terms of community and health care services, there has been general failure of user groups to draw their strength from older users (Means and Lart, 1994a). Ageism and stigma play a part here too, colouring general perceptions of the ability and willingness of older users to participate. Joyce Cormie outlines typical responses to the idea of involving older people in user panels: "They won't be capable of discussing things with you". However, for individual older people there is also a fine balance between recognising the disempowering impact of disability and yet accepting a potentially increasing degree of dependence. The significance of distinguishing between personal and collective empowerment is clear in this instance. For some older people, empowerment may mean handing over tasks which worry them (Stevenson and Parsloe, 1993). Others may feel that their independence is at stake particularly by admitting to problems such as difficulties in running their homes.

There are also implications for the empowerment of older people in the way in which services are delivered. The availability of information about local services may have increased and become more easily accessible due to the efforts of organisations, such as Age Concern, to meet the desire for a 'one-stop shop' for advice (Warren, 1997). Nevertheless, making the most of the system still requires a degree of energy and determination which many frail elderly people may not possess. An additional tension arises from the emphasis in care management on rapid problem identification and prioritisation when older users may need a more exploratory approach and to gain confidence in the agency's ability to offer a relevant service (Hobman, 1994). Substantial numbers of older people have services imposed without consultation, or are 'persuaded' to enter residential care because they are thought to be at risk or their behaviour is socially offensive to others (Allen et al, 1992; Fisher, 1992; Stevenson and Parsloe, 1993). There is little change to the picture post entry: although two thirds of local authorities make regular visits to residential homes, only 13% ask residents for their views on services (Audit Commission, 1993).

Other barriers affecting access to services and communication with 'professionals' include a tendency among older people towards self-effacement; dementia; and researchers' lack of communication skills and knowledge of what it means to be older, as well as their tendency to credit the accounts of other professionals over those of older people themselves (Richards, 1994). Older people are one of the least popular user groups among social workers. Their needs are assumed to be primarily for practical assistance and are therefore seen as less complex and important than those of other users. Subsequently, most social work with older people is carried out by unqualified staff with little understanding or appreciation of the meaning of needs-led assessment (Bland, 1994; Warren, 1997).

Reliance on citizen advocates (Wertheimer, 1993) need not necessarily be the only way to overcoming such barriers to empowerment. As Joyce Cormie's paper demonstrates, the Fife project is an example of how, given adequate transport and meeting facilities, the chance to contextualise their lives and experiences, and control over the agenda of meetings, frail older people can collectively develop their capacity to set their own agenda and speak on their own behalf.

Carers

As potential service users, carers are represented by a relatively strong body of groups, given nationwide publicity by the National Carers' Association and supported, in a number of towns and cities, by Princess Royal Trust-funded Carers' Centres. Carers may also turn to specialist groups such as the Alzheimer's Disease Society and the Relatives' Association for relatives and friends of older people in residential care and nursing homes, as well as numerous local support groups. Some local authorities, for example the Royal Borough of Kingston upon Thames, are appointing Carers' Officers to represent carers' needs (Levick, 1992).

Evidence suggests differences between groups of carers that echo those existing between users. In the Birmingham Community Care Special Action Project (CCSAP) consultation meetings were more positively received by those caring for an older person compared to carers of an adult with a learning disability. It was suggested this may be because the former more 'inexperienced' group were less likely to be in contact with services or carers' networks, while a comparatively well-established lobby of parents of people with learning difficulties already existed in Birmingham. The consultation model was clearly not an appropriate way of making contact with black carers who were seriously under-represented (Barnes and Wistow, 1992c).[6]

At the individual level, it has been argued that the notion of involvement in services is possibly more ambiguous for carers than it is for primary users (Grant, 1992; McGrath and Grant, 1992). Service providers have been identified as conceptualising their relationship with carers in different ways (Twigg, 1989). As 'resources' carers occupy a position that does not fit easily with the expectation that they should play an integral part in service organisation. As 'co-workers', on the other hand, it could be argued that carers would be given a significant role in planning, although the involvement of front-line workers in decision-making processes is still typically limited to immediate day-to-day caring activities only (Walker and Warren, 1996).

There is certainly a tension within community care policy between supporting carers and the central objective of targeting resources on individual service users in greatest need. The latter objective is likely to discriminate against people who have the support of a carer in favour of those who have no one. Evidence shows that, over the past five years, carers have become even less likely to receive any regular help (Henwood, 1993)[7]. Policy also ignores the fact that the majority of carers are women, and has failed to address demands for alternatives which do not exploit women and which give dependent people the right not to rely on their relatives (Finch, 1987). In the case of people with learning difficulties, carers are more likely than users to be involved at all levels – individual, service locality and strategy planning – but this is due to the widespread, and questionable, assumption that they are able to speak on behalf of both their relatives and themselves (Grant, 1992; McGrath and Grant, 1992). There is a clear ethical dimension in the potential conflict between the needs of users and carers, or when user and carer disagree as to what is best for the user, or both (Stevenson and Parsloe, 1993). Yet, at the same time, many carers do not speak out, whatever their viewpoint, for fear that 'rocking the boat' might have damaging consequences – particularly the withdrawal of services – for those for whom they care. From a purely practical perspective, carers looking after people with considerable needs may not have the time or wider support structure to become involved in service organisation on a regular or sustained basis (Warren, 1997).

Community groups

Brian Davey encourages us to consider a notion of empowerment with the potential to bring together all the groups considered so far. Davey's concern is with community empowerment as a way of redeveloping localities 'in crisis'. In his discussion, he draws links between the relationship, health and psychological needs of people and the quality of their environment.

The UK is currently witnessing a rise of 'localism', or the rejection of business and establishment values, as growing coalitions of populist groups oppose government policies, such as the expansion of road building. Greenpeace and Amnesty International are proof that challenges to the prevailing orthodoxy of global development are occurring worldwide. The grassroots cry is rejection of power imposed without consultation or responsibility and demand for a share of resources for all (Vidal, 1995). However, Davey emphasises the fact that the strategy which he advocates cannot be developed at national or international level: it is at the local level that the community has the best understanding of its needs, its human and natural resources and the ways of mobilising those resources.

In terms of welfare, then, Davey calls for a movement away from the pursuit of economic (exogenous) development, which is constrained by the environment and inevitably produces losers, to (endogenous) development focused on communities in their environments. It is an holistic, bottom-up approach, involving the legal enshrinement of people's rights as community members and the development of a general culture of equality. Communities begin to define purposes and agendas for themselves and then to plan, design, implement and monitor their results. The role of local government shifts from initiator to coordinator and supporter of the process, not least through grant aid.

As Davey points out, such models of empowerment have typically been spurned through charges of 'eco-freakishness'. However, the struggle to develop and sustain support for theory born in practice and the experience of powerless communities, rather than in the heads of university academics or extrapolated from professional training manuals, is one common to other disempowered groups. It is a model which is achieving increasing 'official' recognition in the context of policies for regeneration and health improvement (Davies and Kelly, 1993; DoE, Partners in Regeneration, 1995).

Artificial/exclusive boundaries and other qualifications

I have explored the perspectives of a selection of user and carer groups involved in empowering processes but a number of qualifications need to be made before moving on to consider the views of professionals and researchers. The first qualifications relate to the artificiality of categorising participants. It should not be assumed that all users and carers can be placed neatly into one group or another. There are a significant number of service users who fall into more than one category: the commonest overlap is between disabled and older people, though it is not uncommon for people from both groups to be carers too. The factors which impede individual participation in service organisation may therefore be many and complex. On the other hand, people's participation need not necessarily be limited to any one service (Barnes and Wistow, 1992a). Issues of identity aside, bonds could be forged and lessons on overcoming physical barriers and prejudices shared between young people who have had a lifetime's experience of disability and older people who are beginning to face disability at much later stages in their lives (Hobman, 1994). It is worth reflecting here that professionals themselves may also be service users, and that not all disabled people use services.

Another matter to consider is what Stevenson and Parsloe (1993) have termed " 'episodic' incompetence", or what may be more generally referred to as vulnerability. For example, people with a mental illness may vary in their ability to take control of their own lives, although other users may also have periods, when they are in pain and very tired, when the effort required to participate is too much. This is one way in which users' groups come into their own due to their recognition of and ability to sustain members through difficult times.

Alternative ways to explore the experience of users might begin not with disability but with other cross-cutting factors. For example, in terms of health care, people's perspectives on services are likely to be influenced by their relationship to treatment. Williams has defined health service users not simply as those individuals under active treatment, but also those waiting for treatment, believed to need treatment but not seeking it, or not presently receiving treatment but with future treatment needs (Williams, 1985). At a more general level, Taylor et al's discussion of the different terms used to describe users of services leads to an analysis of people's relationship to the separate components of product, service, organisation and State and the subsequent bargaining power they possess (Taylor et al, 1992). Others have highlighted the importance of factors influencing the nature of the relationship between users and services which include voluntariness of user status, length of time of receipt of services, and relationships to others such as carers and citizens in general (Barnes and Wistow, 1992a; Barnes and Prior, 1995).

There are also important distinctions between users which cut across all user groups and may link users to other movements for empowerment. Women are the major users of community care as well as constituting a majority of carers. It is frequently noted that many such women have difficulty in articulating or asserting their needs – especially when they are disabled or of the older generation (Finch, 1990; Douglas, 1992; Stevenson and Parsloe, 1993; Morris, 1994b). Users and carers from black and minority ethnic groups have begun to criticise services for pathologising their behaviour, failing to recognise their specific needs or providing culturally appropriate services, and giving inadequate attention to their significantly different views on illness and experience of racism (Langan, 1990; Atkin, 1991; Squires, 1991; Morton, 1993; Butt, 1994; Warren, 1997).

In sum, the distinct interests of individual users and carers as well as among user and carer groups makes consensus highly unlikely (Barnes and Wistow, 1992a). But, at the same time, focusing upon the specific nature of disability or of the caring relationship encourages a denial of other shared sources of disadvantage and discrimination (Means and Lart, 1994b). It is important to consider the part played by professionals and researchers in exacerbating or ameliorating these situations.

The role of professionals, research and researchers in empowerment

Professionals

All presenters in the seminar series have acknowledged professionals to be more powerful than the individuals with whom they work. Davey observes "the need to reverse the learning relationship". Yet, professionals typically operate within hierarchical, top-down management systems and, as Nina Biehal points out, may themselves lack power to change failings that they perceive in services. Alternatively, they may, as Adrienne Wright found, be genuinely interested in involving users and carers but have limited knowledge and understanding of what involvement might mean and how to extend it. Tensions may therefore be seen to rest on a range of interwoven factors relating to structural obstacles, individual attitudes and expectations, the cultural context in which users receive care and the inadequacy of training and back-up for workers in the introduction of changes to practice.

In practical terms, at one of the most basic levels of giving people a greater individual say in services, assessment measures fail consistently to capture the complexity of individual need. In their attempt to be as comprehensive and sensitive as possible, forms have become long and complex and subsequently are left unused or partially completed (Warren, 1993; Caldock, 1994). Broadening the picture somewhat, experiments in care management have tended to concentrate on defining and costing management tasks. More recent studies of new home care systems, where users are engaged in discussion with providers, show needs still to be responded to in terms of existing provision (Caldock, 1994) and availability of resources: a 'this is what you can pick from' approach (Warren, 1997). While Wright's efforts to shift fellow workers away from the narrow focus on involvement through approaches such as user-satisfaction surveys are a challenge to complacency about current practice, she herself recognises that the framework she developed was still a top-down tool, typical of the health services in as much as it placed emphasis on the 'responsibilities' of professional staff rather than giving precedence to a bottom-up, user perspective.

Professionals may manage these tensions by withholding information. Some social workers appear willing to try a more participatory approach in relatively straightforward cases only: that is, they rule out people suffering from dementia, or deemed at risk or in need of counselling. Alternatively, workers practice 'pseudo-participation': they construct shared records only to accord low priority to user-defined problems and goals (Biehal, 1993), or they resist the need for change by displaying the DATA effect: We Do All This Already (Marsh and Fisher, 1992).

The professional stance which workers adopt is a reflection of the 'peculiar baggage' of concepts, 'practice wisdom', and other information they bring to their jobs (Biehal, 1993). Health service professionals may find it particularly difficult to relinquish their traditionally authoritarian approach (Caldock, 1994). Joyce Cormie's description of the Fife User Panels Project provides vivid illustrations of such resistance from professionals in general. The project determined to place service users – in this case older people – at the centre through their involvement in the advisory group as well as in panel sessions in which they discussed their needs and how they would like them to be met. The aim elicited responses from professionals which included the statement "You don't need to ask them, that is what we are trained to do, we know what all their needs are".

The Fife initiative identified practical factors necessary to secure participation. But equally important was the need for all workers involved in the scheme – the project workers from Age Concern as well as other professionals – to address their own practices by: valuing anecdotal information as an important source of information on older people's backgrounds and attitudes to services; responding to the voice of older people and entering into proactive dialogue rather than attempting to lead with their own agenda; consulting older people on given issues early enough for their opinions to be fed into the planning stage of projects; and freeing themselves of jargon and ageist attitudes. Joyce Cormie's conclusion is that empowerment is not about professionals 'allowing' older people to act differently, but about professionals listening.

However, professionals also need themselves to feel involved in – or to 'own' (Stevenson and Parsloe, 1993) – the processes leading up to change. Studies have confirmed that many workers and first line managers are trying to contribute to the empowerment of users and carers in the face of organisational opposition, explicit or implicit (Stevenson and Parsloe, 1993). In the multi-agency context, the extent of workers' influence over many aspects of user involvement in decision making may be minimal[8]. Disincentives include:

- the short amount of time in which professionals are expected to develop skills and personal values consistent with user and carer empowerment;
- the exclusion of senior managers and front-line staff from training programmes;
- the exclusion of users and carers, both as providers in the programme and as part of the learning group;
- the absence of cross-agency training;
- the adoption of 'plug in' private sector models as the answer to change. (Osborne, 1992; Stevenson and Parsloe, 1993)

Workers may fear losing their role as 'expert'. Supervision is a vital ingredient in breaking down their potential resistance to involving users and in reassuring them of the skills which it demands.

Research and researchers

Questions of how differences between users and professionals are to be captured and, subsequently, to be taken into account in attempts to facilitate and encourage empowerment are increasingly the focus of research. Answering these questions involves the scrutiny of research itself (cf Beresford, 1992; Barnes, 1993, 1995a, 1995b). Grant (1992) has argued that user involvement comes in many forms and, if the impact of empowerment strategies on both service quality and the quality of users' lives is to be teased out, researchers should perhaps be embracing the entire gamut of research designs including longitudinal case studies and experimental design studies. It is not my intention here to address research methodology in the abstract. Rather, I want to consider accounts by researchers of the practice of research and, subsequently, their role in the empowerment process.

The path along which research progresses depends partly upon who decides what matters are examined and how. Those deciding the agenda are unlikely to be researchers alone, but may be a complex amalgam of funders, politicians, professionals and managers. The recent trend within local authority departments of transforming researchers into reviewers and inspectors of services has reduced their power to challenge (Barnes and Wistow, 1992b). Nevertheless, Jabeer Butt (1994) has called for researchers to be honest about the power they are able to exercise in the research setting, admitting that when the research he has conducted has failed to look at issues of disability, it is because he has chosen not to look at them.

From my own experience, I have worked in an institution which relied on income generated by research contracts for its survival. A substantial proportion of those contracts were small-scale, commonly funded by bodies with limited research monies and desirous of instant findings. The combined result was 'fast and dirty' research projects, which offered little prospect of enabling users to have a voice or of contributing to learning about user involvement beyond the level of one-off, semi-structured interviews. Faced with schedules of three to four months in which to conduct and write up research on people with a mental illness about the care management programme, on disabled people attending a day centre about user involvement, and on health professionals about the introduction of service contracts and agreements, I was very much aware of the clash between my personal and academic values and, ultimately, my own economic survival.

In the above instance, the research process was affected primarily by financial resources, with implications for the availability of time. In other situations, time factors are of direct impact. First, there is the sheer length of time it can take for new ideas to become accepted: 'client-oriented' studies have in the past been dismissed as a 'passing fashion' (Davis, 1992, p 33)[9]. The time it takes to carry out purportedly necessary research in an area about which users are campaigning can be used as a substitute for action: responses to user demands are put aside until there are 'findings to discuss' (Davis, 1992, p 40). It is possible that the time lag between 'being involved' and seeing the outcome of that involvement may be a considerable one (Barnes and Wistow, 1992b). Quite often research is unable to benefit those taking part in it and the explicit intention is to benefit future service users (see chapter by Biehal in this volume). Researchers need to draw participants' attention to this. Both parties also need to be aware that failure to review the purpose and guidelines of participatory schemes on a regular basis increases the risk that, over time, involvement will become an end in itself (Grant, 1992).

A final way in which time delays can be of influence may again be illustrated by my own experiences, this time conducting an evaluation of Neighbourhood Support Units (NSUs)[10]. The building of the Support Unit that was to be the original focus of evaluation was delayed – ironically, by a public consultation process – and eventually abandoned. After a year of preparation, the project went into limbo and the coordinator (Hazel Qureshi) left. The project was revived in 1989, six years after its initial conception, but the planned and funded before-and-after experimental evaluation design was rethought and the focus shifted to a Unit already up and running.

The adoption of a pluralistic evaluation model (Smith and Cantley, 1988) – which sought to recognise perceptions of different stakeholders, using semi- and unstructured interviews, group interviews, observation, and time diaries as well as survey questionnaires (Walker and Warren, 1996) – was arguably more fitting than the experimental design for the evaluation of a scheme which aimed to offer greater flexibility and user/carer involvement in service provision. Yet, by this point, other researchers working in the field of health and social care had begun to pursue models which allowed for a far greater degree of user participation. Obversely, when writing up the evaluation, it was important to remember that the NSU initiative was borne on the spring tide of the service user empowerment movement[11] and to avoid falling into the ahistorical trap of judging it according to a standard to which it was not designed to aspire.

Research, then, is the metaphorical onion. It has many layers that often conceal problems not anticipated by researchers. This is perhaps most vividly and honestly demonstrated by Alan France in his discussion of the national evaluation of the role of locally based youth projects in crime prevention.

Here, the research team's proposal to include the views of young people was not resisted by either the project funders (Department for Education) or the steering group, as has commonly been the situation in the past. Problems began to manifest themselves instead when France realised the tightness of the scheduled week-long visits to each of the chosen projects which were intended to comprise meetings and interviews with youth work staff, management and inter-agency partners, as well as informal discussions and observations. Shortages of time simply compounded a variety of other factors hampering the involvement of young people including: the necessity of organising and planning the case studies at a distance; gaining access to young people via youth workers who, guarding their own interests, had in some cases primed participants about their responses to questions; capturing the interest of younger people when it was not clear if they understood what was meant by the evaluation or what France was trying to achieve; and facilitating group sessions when France had no pre-existing relationship with any of the young people and little to offer them in return for their participation, or when younger people did not know each other or feel comfortable talking in groups. Methods which proved more successful in encouraging discussion – such as sitting in on a drugs awareness project meeting – threw up ethical implications related to the degree of choice younger people had exercised in their participation.

France's paper suggests that notions of collaboration were frustrated for both himself, as a researcher, and the young people as participants in the evaluation. If the young people were at all empowered, it was through their refusal to play the researcher's game. The salutary warning is that once research structures are in place it is difficult to alter them and include new methods which, in this case, could have been more rewarding in empowering actors.

The right of users to be heard has featured as a central factor in determining the methods used in other research. Although care leavers had not decided what should be studied, the research team in Nina Biehal's project were committed to involving young people in deciding how the study should proceed and able to do so. The strategies subsequently developed involved care leavers not just as interviewees but also in developing the research questions and commenting on and reviewing the research as it proceeded. Hence, while the research team also felt itself accountable to the local practitioners and managers of the schemes who were included in the project groups, factors aiding participation were identified in a spirit of collaboration rather than conflict or indifference.

Notions of accountability are particularly sharp when research purports to be concerned with the issue of empowerment. There is a potential for individuals to feel 'used' in research (Davis, 1992). Some service users have been deeply affected by the failure to consider their interests as stakeholders: the research process has been described by one member of Survivors Speak Out[12] as "psychiatric pornography" (Mike Lawson cited by Beresford, 1992, p 19). Others feel abandoned when funding runs out and/or is not renewed and relationships which have been carefully built up throughout the duration of a project – particularly if the purpose of that project is advocacy – are suddenly ended (Warren, 1997).

In contrast, Marian Barnes' discussion of the evaluation of the Fife User Panels Project highlights the empowering outcomes of recruiting older people to carry out research, their involvement in which included: adding to the interview schedule; gaining knowledge of and interest in participating in panels; and an increased potential to be more assertive in seeking access to sources of assistance. Nevertheless, Barnes still acknowledges limits in her willingness as a researcher to relinquish control and expertise. She admits to her own lack of confidence in the volunteers' abilities to use unstructured approaches to interviews. As a result of her concern to ensure consistency and comparability, the project therefore employed structured interview schedules. This was despite Barnes' belief that they do not enable responses as rich as those that can be gained from less formal means, and despite the implications for the development of interviewers' skills.

Yet, returning to the wider picture, it is a mistake to assume that all users and carers necessarily want to carry out research themselves. Participants at the workshop did not rank this as a priority in their list of ways forward, preferring, instead, to devote what little spare time they had to tackling their more immediate day-to-day concerns with accessing information, assessment and support which were relevant and sensitive to their needs. And, likewise, while users and carers believed that a key route to achieving these goals was through a better informed health and social care services workforce, and were willing to take part in training sessions, it was not as teachers, per se, but as informants describing their 'personal experiences' and giving their 'perspectives' and 'points of view' (Warren, 1997).

Conclusion

It has been argued that there is no single or correct view on strategies for involvement and little hope of obtaining a consensus about why they are or are not desirable since, in the end, participation is all about politics (Grant, 1992 citing Richardson, 1983).

Certainly, while people are still in what Joyce Cormie described as a 'learning mode', confusion will continue to exist. While I was in the process of writing this paper, *The Guardian* ran a piece on the way in which hospital patients in Devon were finding a voice and using it to improve the training of health service managers. An audio-tape of patients' experiences – developed as part of the training package – had prompted one senior manager to describe himself as having been "slapped around the face for half-an-hour with the truth" (Moore, 1995).

Alliances and partnerships of service users, providers and academics may not be able to come up with *the* definitive meaning of empowerment or *the* successful participatory strategy. What we can aim to do together is (continue to) find ways to rout out the gaps between conceptions of reality construed in terms of varying professional and lay value systems (Grant, 1992); reveal the lived contradictions in policy and their effects on the lives of service users and providers; and boost attempts to promote self-advocacy, including supporting service users to carry out their own research, should this be their desire.

Notes

[1] See, for example, Bradshaw and Gibbs, 1988; Croft and Beresford, 1989, 1990; Walker, 1989, 1992; Percy-Smith and Sanderson, 1992; Taylor et al, 1992; Hoyes et al, 1993; Wistow and Barnes, 1993; Means and Lart, 1994b; Barnes and Walker, 1996; Walker and Warren, 1996; Barnes, 1997.

[2] Living Options has affected local policy in several ways including participation by users and carers in decision making concerning disablement services; surveying services; acting as a watchdog through the drafting of a voluntary code of practice and guidelines on accreditation for private providers,

and through auditing; and through participation in a joint disability forum of senior managers from health, social services, and housing which is chaired by the chairman of the Living Options Working Party.

[3] Commissioned by the Joseph Rowntree Foundation, the Margin to Mainstream project was designed to encourage the development of user- and carer-centred community care through the involvement of users and carers in the planning, management, delivery and quality improvements of local authority services. Sheffield City Council was one of the four sites chosen as case studies for the project.

[4] The Independent Living Fund was a Department of Social Security-funded charity set up in 1988 which paid monthly cash grants to individual disabled people to enable them to buy the help they required directly.

[5] Alan Howarth, MP for Stratford-on-Avon, in a House of Commons debate on disabled people (19 October 1995) reported in *The Guardian*, 'Disabled and denied', 23 October 1995.

[6] It should be noted that CCSAP researchers also concluded that service issues raised during consultation meetings were unlikely to reflect the concerns of carers of people with mental health problems or with physical disabilities, or carers of children with physical or learning disabilities to a similar extent, and that the under-representation of black carers was followed up later.

[7] More than half (55%) of all carers report that the person they are looking after receives no regular visits from either health, social services, or voluntary agencies. Levels of support from social workers, health visitors and, in particular, doctors have all deteriorated.

[8] Hospital social workers noted, for example, that they were sometimes required to set up packages of domiciliary care at such short notice in order to clear beds that exploration of the individual's own views was severely restricted (Biehal, 1993).

[9] Ironically, Davis goes on to observe that, 20 years later on the 'other side' of social work training, students who do not make mention of service users' experiences when writing about their own practice or researching into service provision are given a hard time (Davis, 1992).

[10] Neighbourhood Support Units were a radical initiative developed by Sheffield City Council's Family and Community Services Department with the aim of breaking down the traditional division between domiciliary, day and residential care and to make services more user-oriented with respect to older people and their carers. The first unit, Ecclesfield Elderly Persons Support Unit, was opened in 1985. The evaluation was based on the second unit, which was opened in the Manor area of Sheffield in October 1988 with the new title of Neighbourhood Support Unit (NSU) to reflect its wider use as a community resource.

[11] In policy terms, the NSU initiative was inspired by the Barclay Committee recommendations for a community orientation for social work and emphasis on the importance of informal support networks in the provision of care (Barclay Committee, 1982). It was also underpinned by support for earlier moves towards the decentralisation of social services into small local areas or patches (Hadley and McGrath, 1980; Bayley et al, 1981), although the patch system has since been critiqued as failing to offer people a greater say (Beresford and Croft, 1986).

[12] Survivors Speak Out is the national self-advocacy organisation of people with mental distress.

References

Age Concern (1974) *Manifesto on the place of the retired and elderly in modern society*, London: Age Concern England.

Allen, I., Hogg, D. and Peace, S. (1992) *Elderly people: Choice, participation and satisfaction*, London: Policy Studies Institute.

Atkin, K. (1991) 'Community care in a multi-racial society: incorporating the user view', *Policy & Politics*, vol 19, no 3, pp 159-66.

Audit Commission (1993) *Taking care: Progress with care in the community*, London: HMSO.

Barclay Committee (1982) *Social workers: Their role and tasks*, London: Bedford Square Press.

Barnes, C. and Oliver, M. (1995) 'Disability rights: rhetoric and reality in the UK', *Disability and Society*, vol 10, no 1, pp 111-16.

Barnes, M. (1993) 'Introducing new stakeholders: user and researcher interests in evaluative research. A discussion of methods used to evaluate the Birmingham Community Care Special Action Project', *Policy & Politics*, vol 21, no 1, pp 47-58.

Barnes, M. (1995a) ''Evaluating user and carer involvement in community care'. in J. Waterson and M. Bernard (eds) *Working together: User and carer involvement in community care*, University of Keele: Evaluation Research Unit, pp 12-20.

Barnes, M. (1995b) 'Partnerships in research: working with groups', in G. Wilson (ed) *Community care: Asking the users*, London: Chapman and Hall, pp 228-41.

Barnes, M. (1997) *Care, communities and citizens*, Harlow: Addison Wesley Longman.

Barnes, M., Harrison, S., Mort, S. and Wistow, G. (1996) *Consumerism and citizenship amongst users of health and social care services*, Final Report to the ESRC of Award No L311253025.

Barnes, M. and Prior, D. (1995) 'Spoilt for choice? How consumerism can disempower public service users', *Public Money and Management*, vol 15, no 3, pp 53-8.

Barnes, M. and Walker, A. (1996) 'Consumerism versus empowerment: a principled approach to the involvement of older service users', *Policy & Politics*, vol 24, no 4, pp 375-93.

Barnes, M. and Wistow, G. (1992a) 'Understanding user involvement', in M. Barnes and G. Wistow (eds) *Researching user involvement*, Leeds: Nuffield Institute for Health, University of Leeds, pp 1-15.

Barnes, M. and Wistow, G. (1992b) 'Research and user involvement: contributions to learning and methods', in M. Barnes and G. Wistow (eds) *Researching user involvement*, Leeds: Nuffield Institute for Health, University of Leeds, pp 86-105.

Barnes, M. and Wistow, G. (1992c) 'Consulting with carers: what do they think?', *Social Services Research*, vol 1, pp 9-30.

Bayley, M., Parker, P., Seyd, R. and Tennant, A. (1981) *Neighbourhood services project: Origins, strategy and proposed evaluation*, University of Sheffield: Department of Sociological Studies.

Beresford, P. (1992) 'Researching citizen involvement: a collaborative or colonising exercise?', in M. Barnes and G. Wistow (eds) *Researching user involvement*, Leeds: Nuffield Institute for Health, University of Leeds, pp 16-32.

Beresford, P. and Croft, S. (1986) *Whose welfare: Private care or public services?*, Brighton: The Lewis Cohen Urban Studies Centre, Brighton Polytechnic.

Bewley, C. and Glendinning, C. (1992) *Involving disabled people in community care planning*, York: Joseph Rowntree Foundation.

Biehal, N. (1993) 'Changing practice: participation rights and community care', *British Journal of Social Work*, vol 23, pp 443-58.

Bland, R. (1994) 'EPIC – a Scottish case management experiment', in M. Titterton (ed) *Caring for people in the community: The new welfare*, London and Bristol: Jessica Kingsley, pp 113-29.

Bradshaw, J. and Gibbs, I. (1988) *Public service support for residential care*, Aldershot: Avebury.

Butt, J. (1994) 'Exploring and using the Black resource', *Research, Policy and Planning*, vol 12, no 2, pp 9-12.

Caldock, K. (1994) 'Policy and practice: fundamental contradictions in the conceptualisation of community care for elderly people?', *Health and Social Care*, vol 2, pp 133-41.

Campbell, P. (1993) 'Mental health services – the user's view', in T. Groves (ed) *Countdown to community care*, London: BMJ Publishing Group, pp 105-12.

Croft, S. and Beresford, P. (1989) 'User-involvement, citizenship and social policy', *Critical Social Policy*, vol 26, Autumn, pp 5-18.

Croft, S. and Beresford, P. (1990) *From paternalism to participation: Involving people in social services*, London: Open Services Project and Joseph Rowntree Foundation.

Davies, J.K. and Kelly, M.P. (eds) (1993) *Healthy cities: Research and practice*, London: Routledge.

Davis, A. (1992) 'Who needs user research? Service users as research subjects or participants: implications for user involvement in service contracting', in M. Barnes and G. Wistow (eds) *Researching user involvement*, Leeds: Nuffield Institute for Health, University of Leeds, pp 33-46.

DoE (Department of the Environment)/Partners in Regeneration (1995) *Involving communities in urban and rural regeneration*, London: DoE.

DoH (Department of Health) (1989) *Caring for people: Community care in the next decade and beyond*, London: HMSO.

DoH (1991) *Managers and practitioners: Guide to care management and assessment*, London: HMSO.

Douglas, J. (1992) 'Black women's health matters: putting black women on the research agenda', in H. Roberts (ed) *Women's health matters*, London: Routledge, pp 33-46.

Finch, J. (1987) 'Whose responsibility? Women and the future of family care', in I. Allen, M. Wicks, J. Finch and D. Leat, *Informal care tomorrow*, London: Policy Studies Institute.

Finch, J. (1990) 'The politics of community care in Britain', in C. Ungerson (ed) *Gender and caring: Work and welfare in Britain and Scandinavia*, London: Harvester Wheatsheaf, pp 34-58.

Fisher, M. (ed) (1989) *Client studies*, Sheffield: Joint Unit for Social Services Research.

Fisher, M. (1992) 'Users' experiences of agreements in social care', in M. Barnes and G. Wistow (eds) *Researching user involvement*, Leeds: Nuffield Institute for Health, University of Leeds, pp 47-64.

Goss, S. and Miller, C. (1995) *From margin to mainstream*, York: Joseph Rowntree Foundation.

Grant, G. (1992) 'Researching user and carer involvement in mental handicap services', in M. Barnes and G. Wistow (eds) *Researching user involvement*, Leeds: Nuffield Institute for Health, University of Leeds, pp 65-86.

Hadley, R. and McGrath, M. (eds) (1980) *Going local: Neighbourhood social services*, London: Bedford Square Press.

Henwood, M. (1993) 'What price carers' rights?', *Community Care: Inside Supplement*, 25 March, pp vi-vii.

Hobman, D. (1994) 'What price consumer choice', in Counsel and Care, *More power to our elders: Promoting empowerment for older people,* London: Counsel and Care, pp 1-19.

Hollingberry, R. (1994) 'Elder power', in Counsel and Care, *More power to our elders: Promoting empowerment for older people,* London: Counsel and Care, pp 20-4.

Hoyes, L., Jeffers, S., Lart, R., Means, R. and Taylor, M. (1993) *User empowerment and the reform of community care,* Bristol: SAUS Publications.

Langan, M. (1990) 'Community care in the 1990s', *Critical Social Policy,* vol 29, pp 58-70.

Levick, P. (1992) 'The Janus face of community care legislation: an opportunity for radical possibilities?', *Critical Social Policy,* Issue 34, vol 12, no 1, pp 75-92.

McGrath, M. and Grant, G. (1992) 'Supporting "needs-led" services: implications for planning and management systems (a case study in mental handicap services)', *Journal of Social Policy,* vol 21, no 1, pp 71-97.

Marsh, P. and Fisher, M. (1992) *Good intentions,* York: Joseph Rowntree Foundation with *Community Care.*

Mayer, J.E. and Timms, N. (1970) *The client speaks,* London: Routledge and Kegan Paul.

Means, R. and Lart, R. (1994a) 'Involving older people in community care planning', in Counsel and Care, *More power to our elders: Promoting empowerment for older people,* London: Counsel and Care, pp 25-34.

Means, R. and Lart, R. (1994b) 'User empowerment, older people and the UK reform of community care', in D. Challis, B. Davies and K. Traske (eds) *Community care: New agendas and challenges from the UK and overseas,* Aldershot: Arena, pp 33-43.

Moore, W. (1995) 'Lessons from the bedside', *The Guardian,* 6 December.

Morris, J. (1991) *Pride against prejudice,* London: The Women's Press.

Morris, J. (1994a) 'Community care or independent living?', *Critical Social Policy,* vol 40, pp 24-45.

Morris, J. (1994b) *The shape of things to come: User-led social services,* Social Services Policy Forum Paper No 3, London: National Institute for Social Work.

Morton, J. (ed) (1993) *Recent research on services for black and minority ethnic elderly people*, London: Age Concern.

Oliver, J. (1990) *The politics of disablement*, London: Macmillan.

Osborne, S.P. (1992) 'Lifting the seige? Organisational culture and social services departments', *Local Government Policy Making*, vol 18, no 5, pp 17-20.

Percy-Smith, J. and Sanderson, I. (1992) *Understanding local needs*, London: Institute for Public Policy Research.

Richards, S. (1994) 'Enabling research: elderly people', *Research, Policy and Planning*, vol 12, no 2, pp 5-6.

Richardson, A. (1983) *Participation*, London: Routledge and Kegan Paul.

Simons, K. (1994) 'Enabling research: people with learning difficulties', *Research, Policy and Planning*, vol 12, no 2, pp 4-5.

Smith, G. and Cantley, C. (1988) 'Pluralistic evaluation', in *Evaluation*, Research Highlights in Social Work, 8, London: Jessica Kingsley.

Squires, A. (ed) (1991) *Multicultural health care and rehabilitation of older people*, London: Edward Arnold in association with Age Concern,

Stevenson, O. and Parsloe, P. (1993) *Community care and empowerment*, York: Joseph Rowntree Foundation.

Swain, P. (1993) 'Helping disabled people – the user's view', in T. Groves (ed) *Countdown to community care*, London: BMJ Publishing Group, pp 96-104.

Taylor, M., Hoyes, L., Lart, R. and Means, R. (1992) *User empowerment in community care: Unravelling the issues*, DQM 11, Bristol: SAUS Publications.

Twigg, J. (1989) 'Models of carers: how do agencies conceptualise their relation with informal carers?', *Journal of Social Policy*, vol 18, no 1, pp 43-66.

Vidal, J. (1995) 'Localism vs globalism', an edited and amended version of an article published in *The printer's devil*, November, in *The Guardian*, 15 November.

Walker, A. (1989) 'Community care', in M. McCarthy (ed) *The new politics of welfare*, London: Macmillan, pp 203-24.

Walker, A. (1992) 'Increasing user involvement in the social services', in T. Arie (ed) *Recent advances in psychogeriatrics 2*, London: Churchill Livingstone, pp 5-9.

Walker, A. and Warren, L. (1996) *Changing service for older people: The Neighbourhood Support Units innovation*, Buckingham: Open University Press.

Warren, L. (1993) 'Community care and user participation', in P. Kaim-Caudle, J. Keithley and A. Mullender (eds) *Aspects of ageing: A celebration of the European Year of Older People and Solidarity Between Generations 1993*, London: Whiting and Birch Ltd, pp 127-39.

Warren, L. (1997) *Alliances and partnerships in empowerment: The 'Working in Partnership' Workshop*, Unpublished report, Sheffield: Department of Sociological Studies, University of Sheffield.

Wertheimer, A. (1993) *Speaking out. Citizen advocacy and older people*, Report No 19, London: Centre for Policy on Ageing.

Whittaker, A. (1990) 'Involving people with learning difficulties in meetings', in L. Winn (ed) *Power to the people: The key to responsive services in health and social care*, London, King's Fund Centre for Health Services, pp 41-8.

Williams, A. (1985) *Medical ethics: Health service efficiency and clinical freedom*, Nuffield/York Portfolios, No 2, York: York University.

Wistow, G. and Barnes, M. (1993) 'User involvement in community care: origins, purposes and applications', *Public Administration*, Autumn.